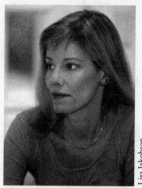
Lisa Jakobson

About the Author

CATHRYN JAKOBSON RAMIN is an investigative journalist who has written for many national publications, including the *New York Times Magazine* and *O, The Oprah Magazine*. She lives with her husband, film composer Ron Ramin, and two teenage sons in northern California. She is a fellow of the MacDowell Colony, as well as a member of the National Association of Science Writers and the San Francisco Writers' Grotto. She is the founder of Managing the Midlife Mind, an organization that helps corporations support the cognitive needs of their older employees. This is her first book.

CARVED
IN SAND

· · ·

CATHRYN JAKOBSON RAMIN

· · ·

CARVED IN SAND

When Attention Fails
and Memory Fades in Midlife

· · ·

HARPER

NEW YORK · LONDON · TORONTO · SYDNEY

HARPER

"Forgetfulness" from *Questions About Angels*, by Billy Collins © 1991. Reprinted with the permission of the University of Pittsburgh Press.

To protect privacy, many names of contributors to this book have been changed. Anonymous individuals are referred to by a single first name. When a given name and a surname appear, it is the actual name of a person.

I am not a physician or a psychologist, and therefore nothing in this book should be interpreted as medical or psychological advice. No treatments or therapies should be undertaken without consulting a physician or mental health professional.

A hardcover edition of this book was published in 2007 by HarperCollins Publishers.

FIRST HARPER PAPERBACK PUBLISHED 2008.

Designed by Kathryn Parise

Library of Congress Cataloging-in-Publication Data is available upon request.

ISBN: 978-0-06-059870-9 (pbk.)

08 09 10 11 12   ID/RRD   10 9 8 7 6 5 4 3 2 1

To Ron, Avery and Oliver . . . memories are made of this

CONTENTS

. . .

Forgetfulness

The name of the author is the first to go
followed obediently by the title, the plot,
the heartbreaking conclusion, the entire novel
which suddenly becomes one you have never read,
never even heard of,

as if, one by one, the memories you used to harbor
decided to retire to the southern hemisphere of the brain,
to a little fishing village where there are no phones.

Long ago you kissed the names of the nine Muses goodbye
and watched the quadratic equation pack its bag,
and even now as you memorize the order of the planets,

something else is slipping away, a state flower perhaps,
the address of an uncle, the capital of Paraguay.

Whatever it is you are struggling to remember,
it is not poised on the tip of your tongue,
not even lurking in some obscure corner of your spleen.

It has floated away down a dark mythological river
whose name begins with an L as far as you can recall,
well on your own way to oblivion where you will join those
who have even forgotten how to swim and how to ride a bicycle.

No wonder you rise in the middle of the night
to look up the date of a famous battle in a book on war.
No wonder the moon in the window seems to have drifted
out of a love poem that you used to know by heart.

—Billy Collins

PREFACE

. . .

Most Precious Possession

There was no way around it. Something was happening to my mind. I felt vague and foggy. I couldn't remember what I'd read for much longer than it took to get to the bottom of the page. Almost overnight, I found that I was missing critical information—the names of people and places, the titles of books and movies. Words, my stock-in-trade as a writer, had started to play hide-and-seek. Thoughts popped in and out of my mind, barely formed, so evanescent that even when I dashed for paper and pencil, I didn't have time to record them. My mental calendar, once easily summoned, grew elusive and developed blank spots, as did my sense of direction. My life became billowy, amorphous, as if someone had removed the support poles from my tent. The change was so dramatic that sometimes I felt foreign to myself.

I'd barely crossed the threshold of middle age. It was a bad time, made worse because I was afraid to tell anyone what had befallen me. I didn't have the words to describe it, or the heart to contend with the solicitous expressions I expected to encounter if I spoke up. Whatever this was, it was mine alone. As a journalist, I was invested in staying smart and quick, mistress of my good brain and my sardonic tongue.

Secretly, I assumed that I had lost my edge, a ruinous thing in my business. I had a lovely husband and two beautiful young sons. As rich as those blessings made me, my identity and my self-esteem depended on the quality of my thinking.

A chance conversation with a fifty-year-old friend, one of the sharpest women I know, made me realize that I was not alone. One morning, over coffee, she explained that she was quitting her job. She had suffered a string of frightening moments, when her mind emptied as quickly as the shoreline before a tsunami, leaving her feeling, as she put it, "like an old fool." I'd seen my aunt hold up two index fingers, close her eyes, and ask me to wait while she worked her way through a "senior moment," but as far as I was concerned, such lapses were the exclusive domain of people who were much older.

"My memory is shot," my friend muttered. "It could be stress, or depression, or insomnia, or menopause, or that I hate my job, or that I was crazy to wait until I was forty-four to have a child. What I know is that I'm working with people who are twenty-five years younger than I am and they will not cut me any slack. I don't know how bad it will get, or how it will end, but I'll tell you one thing: I'd rather die than lose my mind."

Within a few weeks, she stopped working and started taking Zoloft: Her psychiatrist was convinced that depression was to blame for her memory troubles. Although depression is often a catalyst for midlife memory impairment, it is not the only cause. Worth considering is the converse: The apparently sudden onset of cognitive troubles—with onerous implications in terms of aging and professional success—could be harrowing enough to bring it on. I could no longer visit her in the midafternoon because she required a long daily nap. I watched her previously robust self-confidence disappear as her world contracted.

Soon after, I went to the movies with my husband. On the short drive home, I realized that I couldn't remember the title of the film, which I had liked very much, or the name of the actor who played the leading role. For some reason, this was the last straw. It shook me up. The bulldozer that had run over my friend was already rolling in my direction. I wasn't going to lie down for it. If there was some way to fight these alterations in memory and attention, to snatch my brain out of harm's way, I'd summon the gumption, and I'd fight.

I began with the self-help books, of which there were many, each of which promised that (with a little work) I could capture forever the names of people I met at cocktail parties. Presumably intended for an older audience with a good deal of armchair time at its disposal, the books bored and frustrated me. I found it difficult to remember their "tips and tricks," and impossible to pay sufficient attention to the brainteasers to solve them. I struggled through the diagnostic quizzes that populated the pages of the self-help books, feeling that they weren't intended for my demographic. I filled out multiple-choice tests that asked how often I hunted for missing items—never, once a week, every other day or once a day, or multiple times a day. Who were they kidding? People in their forties (and many in their fifties) were still in the stage of life where, in the course of an hour, they'd need to track down sneakers, missing homework assignments, a single green sock and a stuffed animal. Add those to the search for the missing car keys, the elusive digital file, the shopping list and the lunch meat, and life became a perpetual treasure hunt. No wonder people were obsessed with "getting organized." The aisles of the Container Store, the newest behemoth in our local mall, were filled with middle-aged people determined to get a grip on their lives.

Over the course of a few years, as many of my friends and relatives moved into their forties and fifties, I began to realize that actually, I was part of a large group of middle-aged people who were struggling to keep up. When Sol Wisenberg, then the government counsel, asked former president Bill Clinton to repeat the details of an exchange he'd had eight months earlier with Vernon Jordan, regarding Monica Lewinsky, the fifty-two-year-old Clinton said that he couldn't remember. To many, it sounded like a convenient excuse, but not to me. I believed him. Why should he be different from anybody else? In *The Starr Report,* published in 1998, he was uncharacteristically forthcoming: "If I could say one thing about my memory," he told Wisenberg, ". . . I have been shocked and so have members of my family and friends of mine at how many things I have forgotten in the last six years—I think because of the pressure and pace and volume of events in a president's life . . . I'm amazed—there are a lot of times that I literally cannot remember what happened last week."

Everywhere I went, I noticed that people's conversations had begun to resemble the game of charades, where all they could produce were fractional notions of what they wanted to say—"sounds like . . . starts with . . . three syllables." A handsome fiftyish waiter at one of the finer restaurants in the Napa Valley, a pro who took his job seriously, forgot one of our appetizers, and then one of our desserts, at which point he became so apologetic that I thought he was about to cry. When Pixar brought out the animated film, *Finding Nemo*, a movie that involved, among other characters, a very forgetful middle-aged fish named Dory, a handy new code word was born. "Dory," one woman would say sharply to another, warning her that she had commenced to tell, yet again, a story she had told days—or even hours—before. It seemed that I had plenty of company, both male and female.

"It's like this," one woman said, describing the extended wait she experienced when she tried to bring information to mind. "I used to have the *Jeopardy* answers long before the buzzer. I still know them, but I just can't find them as fast. I'm no longer an AK-47. I'm more like a musket; you've got to load it, tamp it, pack it down and then fire."

I was determined to get a plausible explanation of what was happening to my brain, and by extension, to middle-aged minds in general. My forgetfulness was running my life. Was this normal aging? Was it something else? I could either give up, resigning myself to existence in a mental fog, or I could subject my brain to the best scientific analysis and medical treatment.

I saw my opening and I took it. I'd become a guinea pig, a self-appointed representative of middle-aged people whose brains were behaving unnervingly. I'd seek interventions of all kinds, from established to fringe, because who knew where the answer might be found? This sort of interior exploration carried risks, both pharmacological and intellectual, but the way I saw it, I had little choice. I'd consult with a range of experts in many disciplines, from bench scientists who worked primarily with animals and microscopes to the first generation of clinicians who had ready access to the human brain in vivo, thanks to the availability of MRI and PET brain-scanning technology. Before I was through, I'd meet with cognitive psychologists, psychiatrists, neuropsychologists, neurologists, neuroscientists, sleep-medicine specialists, pharmacologists, gerontologists, geneticists, trauma experts, toxicologists, endocrinologists and nutritionists. For good measure, I'd throw in a guru or two. There were obvious flaws in my methodology: No self-respecting scientist would design an investigation that allowed multiple research protocols to occur simultaneously. But I wasn't a scientist. I was a journalist who knew a good story when I saw one. Forgetfulness was on all of our minds. It was driving us nuts. And I was going to get us some answers.

At the very beginning of my research, I wrote to Gary Small, an esteemed psychiatrist who directs both the UCLA Center on Aging and the UCLA Memory Clinic. In four pages, I outlined my memory difficulties, explaining that I had been commissioned to write an article on the subject of midlife forgetfulness for the *New York Times Magazine*, and that eventually, that article would grow into a book. To be honest, I expected to get a form letter back, telling me that he didn't see patients. Instead, he phoned and offered me the moon—a full evaluation, including a trip through the PET scanner and the MRI machine. In terms of memory evaluation, this was the gold standard. I was on my way.

Every time I mentioned my plans for this book—in a doctor's reception area, in the hair salon, while I stood waiting in high winds for a bus—I was treated to a discourse that left me scribbling on purse-worn grocery lists. Once I promised that I'd maintain their anonymity (and that was critical; many individuals were extremely nervous about "coming out"), people made me privy to their own stories. Some are sad, and some are hilariously funny. I never intended to write a self-help book or an impenetrable scientific treatise. Instead, this book dwells in the realms of forgetfulness-fraught reality, peppered with the perspectives of middle-aged individuals from many walks of life. There is Daniel, normally meticulous in his actions, who forgot that he was wearing a lined raincoat and slipped his passport between the layer of poplin and the layer of wool, whereupon it promptly fell to the floor in the Zurich airport, unnoticed by him. There is Wendy, who lost her key card, and let herself into the wrong hotel room after convincing the housekeeping staff to open the door. There is Charlie, the lawyer who packed his bag before heading out of town for an important case, only to discover that he had to muster his courtroom defense in wrinkled chinos, having left his suit pants behind. Just as I have, I feel sure that you, the reader, will find comfort in the knowledge that you are part of a community, one that I came to call "the memory-hungry crowd."

Given the limitations of my memory, it did not take me long to realize that I needed a more systematic and reliable method of recording people's thoughts. I developed a survey, ten pages long. Though I sent out hundreds by e-mail and snail mail, I feared that people would toss my questions in the trash, unanswered. I was wrong. Apparently, many had been waiting for this opportunity. Answering was time-consuming, but also cathartic. People asked me for permission to send the survey to sisters-in-law and old college roommates. It was viral, in a good way. A group of nurses in Georgia got hold of it, as did a bevy of school administrators in Milwaukee. It found its way to a cluster of retired air-traffic controllers (all-but-mandatory retirement age: fifty-six) and then to a bunch of JetBlue employees. Briefly, it infiltrated the sales force in the sportswear department of Neiman Marcus in Boston, and a police officers' association in the Bronx. It had a brief run with some bus drivers in Raleigh-Durham after I watched one of them receive a dressing-down from his very irritated girlfriend because he'd forgotten their plans for a church picnic. I never knew where it would turn up next. In the end, I collected data from more than two hundred people, from Texas to Timbuktu, over a period of two years. In nearly every instance, my correspondents carefully checked the box on the survey requesting that they maintain anonymity. I found that very interesting. People who were willing to air their views about virtually any other subject were determined to keep their forgetfulness under wraps. I understood, of course—I'd struggled with the same feelings. Admit forthrightly to a disturbing level of memory loss and you could expect to watch your clients and constituents flee in horror.

Once, I pushed too hard. One woman, a senior marketing executive who was extremely forthcoming about the freight train that hit her at fifty, turned jittery when I began eliciting details that she thought might identify her to her employees. It was simply too risky.

Such reticence was rare, however. After my correspondents returned the survey, they often remained in touch, checking in regularly to ask how I was doing, and when the book would be ready. I should be sure, they wrote, to include information about a never-ending list of topics, including stress, insomnia, diet, trauma, menopause, anxiety, depression, toxic exposure, substance abuse, attention-deficit disorder and Alzheimer's disease.

The same questions kept surfacing: Why does forgetfulness scare the pants off us? Is your memory something you inherit, like your eye color? How can you hang on to what you have left? Is there some way to get back what you have already lost? Could something you did way back in your misspent youth affect your brain in middle age? Is menopause to blame for your forgetfulness? Were there pills you could take to improve your memory? Were there exercises you could do? Was there some way to protect yourself from Alzheimer's disease, which these days seems to lurk in every family?

There were endless questions, but to me, this seemed like the most pressing: What allows some people to maintain their faculties well into old age, while their peers struggle? One day, I was walking the dogs at sunrise, on a bike path that ran along a nearby creek. I was enjoying a full forty-five minutes with nothing to do while I waited for my son to finish his session with his math tutor, when I spotted a sinewy older man with an unusual gait. Every few running strides, he lurched forward, then caught himself and continued on his way. On each knee, just below the hem of his form-fitting Lycra athletic shorts, he'd wrapped an Ace elastic brace, the kind you buy at the drugstore. He caught up to me quickly, adjusted the angle of his light blue fishing hat and introduced himself as Zvi Danenberg. He was eighty years old, and he jogged between eight and fifteen miles a day, depending on the weather. He'd run nearly eighty thousand miles in his life, in his own estimation, all of them since he'd turned sixty-five, when the doctor recommended long, slow walks for a sore lower back. "To tell you the truth," he said, in an old-country accent, "this walking, it bored me silly. So one day, I ran a hundred yards, just to break things up, and that was it. I was hooked."

He was in excellent physical shape for his age, but what was really important about running, he confided, was the social life it engendered. It helped keep his brain in trim. "I know the names of two hundred and fifty people and dogs and some cats, too, that I meet on this walking path," he said, after ascertaining that the shepherd mutt sitting politely beside me was Rosie, and that Radar was the little Havanese who was frantically trying to climb his leg. "And you," he said, as if he were cementing the knowledge in his mind, "are Cathryn." By now, the sun was up and every few yards along the path, we stopped to greet another jogger or dog walker. He took pains to introduce me to everyone.

"Running is only one of my interests," Zvi announced, as we moved along at a good clip. Music was his true love. He had a collection of nineteen thousand LPs and five thousand compact discs, embracing a range of classical and world music, and the numbers were still growing. If I'd like, I could see the collection. He could put his hand on just about any album he wanted, in a matter of seconds.

"How do you know how many LPs you have?" I asked.

"I was a high school math and physics teacher for thirty years," he said. "Numbers and facts stick to me like glue. But I'm nothing much. I should introduce you to some of my friends." He nodded to Sam, ninety-three, who was just then speed-walking in our direction.

Zvi hadn't been physically active in middle age; with his teaching job, he hadn't found the time. When he retired, and stopped doing math and physics every day, his mind began to slacken as quickly as his unused abdominal muscles. Instead of giving in to a slower, more muddled existence, he kicked it up a notch, resolutely refusing to make the excuses that come so readily with the years. He ran in any weather—in the last decade, the only thing that had stopped him, he said, "was a temperature of a hundred and three." He kept company with a lively bunch of pals, none of whom were inclined to sit around and watch TV. A few times a week he ventured to the East Bay to attend a concert, sometimes with a friend but often on his own, or he took the bus to San Francisco's Symphony Hall to sit in on the pre-concert lectures. Like the enthusiastic student he is, Zvi was the one with his hand raised at the end. In the last third of his life, he'd pursued new passions. When he talked about them, his craggy face lighted up and his blue eyes sparkled.

In Zvi, I discovered hope for all of us. But hope wasn't enough. I needed answers. This book chronicles my journey in pursuit of an agile brain that could carry me smartly through midlife and into my old age. For over two years, I traveled, meeting specialists and interviewing experts. I spent far too many nights in hotel rooms with polyester bedspreads. But here's the funny thing: I never felt alone, not for a minute. The memory-hungry crowd was with me, even when I had my head in the PET scanner. The answers I found are for all of us. Although the details of midlife forgetfulness may vary from person to person, ultimately, we're all in the same boat. If you've been a member of the memory-hungry crowd for a while now, thanks for coming along for the ride. If you've only just joined us, welcome. You're in good company, and I'm delighted to tell you that you're *finally* going to find out exactly what's going on upstairs.

CARVED
IN SAND

. . .

1

YOUR UNRELIABLE BRAIN

. . .

Midlife Forgetfulness Is Embarrassing and Frustrating, but What Does It Mean for the Future?

On the drive from the suburbs to the city, we'd experienced a disturbing number of memory lapses. Actually, the first bout with forgetfulness had occurred earlier that afternoon, when our friend Sam, who was three hours away in Reno judging a barbecue contest, forgot that we had dinner plans. After a not-so-gentle phone reminder from his wife, he made the drive home in record time, still carrying a whiff of slow-smoked baby back ribs on his person. That mistake was in the past, but other canyons loomed before us. Where was our restaurant, again? (I had printed out the address, as I'd promised—and left it on the kitchen counter.) Had my husband made the reservation for seven, or seven-fifteen? Which way did Post Street go? Was the nearest parking lot on the corner, or midway up the block? I made the error of mentioning that the little bistro we'd chosen had a great young chef, fresh out of the kitchen of some hotshot who had a restaurant in the Napa Valley, and another in Los Angeles. Or maybe it was Las Vegas. I'd read about it somewhere.

That's what set my husband off.

"Oh, I know exactly who you mean," he said, ready to educate us. Then, he drew a blank. I watched him become increasingly preoccupied as he explored every shadowy cognitive pathway, searching for the name he was after.

I whispered that he ought to give it a rest—he'd think of it later.

"But it's driving me crazy," he said.

An hour into this hard-earned evening out with friends, more information was missing than present. Among our peers, this state of affairs was so common I'd started to call it "the content-less conversation." When the words "Ken Frank, La Toque, Fenix—and that *is* in L.A." finally tumbled from his lips, we cheered. We could move on to other things, like whether any of us had ever tasted the nice bottle of wine we were ordering, and if we had, whether we'd liked it. Maybe we'd only heard about it. Or read about it. Or seen it on the supermarket shelf. No one could say for sure.

"I guess this is normal," Julia sighed, "but I swear, no one we know can remember a thing."

"It may be normal," Sam said darkly, "but it isn't acceptable. Maybe forty years ago, when life was slower and you could depend on a pension and a gold watch for thirty years of dedicated service, it would have been okay."

He was right: What was making us nuts hadn't flustered our parents in their forties and fifties. But their lives were different, and so were their expectations. They weren't changing careers or inventing new ones. At the age of fifty-two, they definitely weren't trying to remember to show up for back-to-school night for three kids at two different schools.

NORMAL—BUT NOT ACCEPTABLE

Nearly every time the subject of forgetfulness arose, people asked me if what they were experiencing was "normal." If they defined that word as the dictionary does—"conforming with, adhering to, or constituting a norm, standard, pattern, level or type," the answer was yes—perfectly.

Everybody asked, but in truth, few people were content with the implications of "normal." What they really wanted to know was whether they were just a little (or a lot) better off than their peers. This was important: If they slipped below the mean, chances were good that they would not be able to keep up.

What was normal had changed considerably over the centuries: Two hundred years ago, if we aged "normally"—that is, according to our biological destiny—forgetfulness wouldn't be an issue at forty-five or fifty: Most of us would be in our graves. Medicine constantly redefines what is normal in terms of physiological aging. We get new knees and new hips. We take drugs to control our blood pressure. We don't give up reading when our fading vision demands that we hold the newspaper at arm's length. Instead, we build ourselves an arsenal of reading glasses and scatter them all over the house and office, in case we forget where they are. When the *New York Times Magazine* began to run a Sunday cartoon series with wording in a font so small that I couldn't manage it even while wearing my reading glasses, I suffered no damage to my self-esteem. And yet, when it comes to what scientists call "age-associated cognitive impairment," we take it personally and refuse to do anything about it, mostly because we're not sure what we *can* do.

This sheeplike complacency occurs because the brain is our most intimidating organ. Your brain, with you from the start, has demanded remarkably little attention. Like me, you've probably spent more time worrying about the condition of your abdominal muscles. We assume that what is going on in there is as mysterious as the universe, involving such concepts as consciousness, being and soul, surely best left to the philosophers and the clerics. Here's the news: From a purely biochemical perspective, your brain—a three-pound bolus of fat, with the texture of lightly scrambled eggs—is essentially the same organ a rat is carrying around on its shoulders. As a result of your genetic inheritance, certain aspects of how your brain will age are already inscribed in the *Book of You*, but it's written in pencil, and you have an eraser. Recent studies of pairs of elderly identical twins, only one of whom developed Alzheimer's disease, show that genetics, although influential, aren't everything. As you will see, you can indeed influence the way your brain ages, through diet, physical and mental exercise, and assuming you've done all you can in those departments, by taking advantage of the increasing availability of pharmaceuticals intended to enhance cognition.

Say it to yourself: "Normal, but not acceptable." And, from what the senior scientists tell me, definitely mutable, subject to the quality of your resolve.

I'll wager that when presbyopia set in, some time in your forties, and you could no longer read the small print, you didn't tell yourself that if you only tried harder, you could conquer your farsightedness, nor did you ruminate about hiding your deficiency from your friends, family and employers.

Not so when your memory began to fail, you suddenly had the attention span of a flea and you felt like you were moving in slo-mo through cognitive Jell-O. In *that*, there was a portentousness: Maybe the foundation of your existence was crumbling and this was the beginning of the end. For people who have always been very competent, with a talent for thinking on their feet, forgetting brings a disturbing sense of the loss of control and mastery.

"Memory loss is a stealth killer," said Peggy, a corporate consultant. For years, her quick mind and her sharp wit were her calling cards. Companies hired her because she was a very fast study, able to march into a corporate boardroom, absorb quantities of unfamiliar data, assess the holes in a strategy and produce a new, improved one, fast. It's getting a lot harder, she said. "There are a million ways I know my brain is different. It's managed, in a few short years, to rob me of my pride and self-esteem. I notice that the 'ah-ha' moments of insight, on which I rely, are fewer, and frankly, they yield less fruit."

People who glided through their school days and early professional years blessed with nearly encyclopedic recall and the ability to keep multiple plates spinning in the air, who've never relied on calendars or kept meticulous notes, suffer the most. "I used to be able to do it all almost flawlessly," said Rudy, who runs a manufacturing company. "It was all up here," he said, pointing to his bald pate, "but recently I've started to cross wires." Predictably, he blew a circuit. He sent off a new manual to be printed and bound—100,000 copies—failing to indicate the location of a critical switch. The new equipment, fresh from the factory, piled up in the warehouse, while the corrected manual was reprinted, at considerable expense. No one got paid for a long time, and he acknowledged that his error could have tanked the company. "It could not have happened before," he said, "and I find it terrifying."

It may seem as if midlife forgetfulness arrives overnight. "One day I was fine," acknowledged Laura, the marketing manager of a retail company. "Better than fine, really. I was a whiz. And the next day, I was struggling to remember the names of the people who work for me." In fact, the decaying of memory and attention is a slow process that begins in our twenties, when we start to lose processing speed. (Mice, rats and primates experience the same decline.) Because you're endowed with redundant systems—enough spare neurons to get you through—you don't feel it right away. By the time you reach your early forties, however, there are significant differences from the early-to-mid-twenties peak—and it's essentially downhill from there.

"It's not the fact of the memory deficit that's the problem," avowed clinical psychologist Harriet Lerner, author of *The Dance of Anger*, when I asked her what she thought lay beneath the surface. "It's the anxiety that comes with it. Forgetting becomes globalized. It's no longer about the file you can't find on your desk. Now it's about the prospect of rapid mental deterioration. You interpret your latest error to mean that you're on a fast, deep slope to aging, perhaps faster than your best friend or your colleague, and that you will shortly be revealed as inadequate, unworthy, unintelligent and undesirable company for the people who pay your salary, as well as the ones you love and respect. Not surprisingly, that's when the fear and shame kick in."

The more anxious you become, Lerner explained, the more likely you are to ruminate, an activity that is guaranteed to make matters worse. "People become overfocused, in an obsessive, nonproductive way," she said. "You start waking up at three in the morning, catastrophizing about what you've forgotten. You begin to avoid circumstances where your weakness will be revealed—staying out of conversations and backing away from work challenges, for instance. But avoidance doesn't work. It only makes the shame grow."

When you start that slide into shame and fear, it's difficult to put on the brakes. You lose access to higher-level reasoning, the aspect of thinking that allows you to say, "Hey, maybe you're making a mountain out of a molehill." Instead, the primitive brain takes over and you plummet into a black-and-white thinking, where subtle differences don't exist. When shame and fear arise—even if it's because you can't remember your ATM password—the primitive brain takes you straight into survival mode. It says, "Hey, buddy, you could be in deep trouble here." Suddenly, this is not about your password. It's not even about feeling foolish as you hold up the Friday afternoon line at the cash machine. It's about your ability to do your job, to manage your life, to remain safe, to feed yourself and your family and to keep a roof over your head.

WHAT DOES THE FUTURE HOLD?

Our forgetfulness is fraught with implications about who we will become as we age. It's easy to allow feelings of embarrassment, frustration and anger to plunge us into fear—cold, implacable anxiety emerging from the suspicion that we might have decades of dependence ahead of us, with a diminished mind trapped in a still vigorous body.

Without question, the people who worry about it the most are the ones who have had the misfortune of watching a loved one decline into Alzheimer's disease. Today, that experience is common: Alzheimer's occurs in 35 percent of people eighty and older. Of the two hundred individuals who replied to my survey, more than one-third had watched a first-degree relative—parent, aunt or uncle—fall into Alzheimers' grip. Understandably, they began to observe themselves closely. "After watching my mother lose her memory to Alzheimer's, I am hypersensitive to every little memory slip," said Evelyn, a singer and songwriter. "The other day, I couldn't remember the name of a business acquaintance I wanted to introduce to my husband at the supermarket. She wound up introducing herself, very pointedly, and I felt as if I'd not only insulted her, but that I'd failed in some profound way."

Washington Post columnist George Will explained what it was like to watch the disease take hold of his mother. "Dementia is an ever-deepening advance of wintry whiteness," he wrote, "a protracted paring away of personality. It inflicts on victims the terror of attenuated personhood.... No one has come back from deep in that foreign country to report on life there. However, it must be unbearably frightening to feel one's self become as light as a feather, with inner gales rising."

I met Phyllis in Weymouth, Massachusetts, at an Alzheimer's clinic. She'd brought her seventy-two-year-old mother, Margaret, to be evaluated. I stood in a niche between the door and the exam table, a fly on the wall as Margaret's new physician asked her questions. She didn't know what floor of the building she was on, but she knew which county she stood in. He offered her three words—"ball, flag and tree"—and then asked her to repeat them a few minutes later. Even with coaching, she could not. He asked her to draw a clock, with the hands placed at ten after eleven, but it was not possible.

During the exam, I watched Phyllis's face. She wore a slight smile, meant, I expect, to comfort her mother, who had no idea why her daughter insisted on this visit. When the doctor offered his assessment—Margaret was about to enter stage two of Alzheimer's, when the disease usually took off like wildfire—the patient continued to sit placidly on the table, swinging her legs, but Phyllis started to cry. Margaret would need to stop driving right away, the doctor said, and it would be a good idea to switch the gas stove in her kitchen for an electric one.

"You're taking away her independence," Phyllis said. "She'll be horrified." I could see the fear clutching at her. She was grieving, of course, for her mother. But there was more to it: Phyllis was considering her own prospects. Nothing scares us more than the thought of becoming someone else's burden.

In the waiting room, Phyllis confided in me. It wasn't the right thing to be thinking about, she told me, not when her mother was in such trouble. But she wondered if I could tell her something. In the last few years, she'd noticed changes in her memory—nothing big, for sure—but enough to set her on her heels. Did her own lapses mean that in twenty-five years, or even less, she'd wind up like her mother?

I knew very well what she wanted me to say: that what she was experiencing was normal; that midlife memory failures, as irritating as they are, signify nothing; that these small incidences of forgetfulness are not evidence of a trickling stream of damage that would eventually grow into a torrent, and devastate memory, language and reason.

In good faith, I couldn't tell Phyllis what she wanted to hear. Every day, a new study rolls out of a university lab confirming that Alzheimer's isn't a disease that suddenly rears its head in old age. Current research shows that decades before clinical symptoms arise—in middle age or even before—the seeds of Alzheimer's disease are already planted. To insist otherwise is to indulge in the most unhealthy sort of denial. Her symptoms could be portentous—or might mean that her middle-aged brain was simply overcome with the responsibilities of working, caring for her children and taking care of her declining mother.

Today, 4.5 million Americans have Alzheimer's disease. It's the eighth leading cause of death in the United States, and nearly as prevalent in

Japan and Europe. In 2005, Alzheimer's cost the federal government $91 billion in Medicare costs. By 2010, that number will be closer to $160 billion. If the disease proceeds unimpeded, in twenty years the number of people with Alzheimer's is projected to increase to fourteen million. When you consider that by 2030, almost one in five Americans will be over sixty-five, it is apparent that we face a public health burden that will swamp us.

"By the time even the earliest symptoms of Alzheimer's are detectable by clinicians," explained John C. Morris, director of the Center for Aging at Washington University, "there is already substantial brain damage, actual cell loss, in the critical areas of learning and attention. There is little or nothing that science can do to restore those neurons to their original state. We need to start tracking forty-year-olds. You don't want to wait until you have to say to somebody, 'Your PET scan just lit up like a Christmas tree.'"

The goal of nearly every Alzheimer's researcher is to find a way to identify the beginning of the disease process. "If we can meet this disease in the earliest stage, and counteract it with drugs that reverse the damage, science would no longer be in the position of trying to build new neurons," said John Q. Trojanowski, director of the Penn Institute on Aging and Alzheimer's Disease at the University of Pennsylvania. "It is in your forties, or maybe even younger, that normal memory loss begins to diverge from pathological memory loss. In my lab, we're spending a lot of time trying to define that fork in the road, where you either continue to lose a little bit of your memory capacity each year, and remain essentially normal, or you take the other fork, where you are on a downward trajectory, culminating in dementia."

What sparks Alzheimer's disease? Attend an international Alzheimer's meeting, as I did in Philadelphia, and you will quickly realize, as you mill around with five thousand scientists, that for every hypothesis, there's a contradictory one. Read the peer-reviewed journals, however, and you'll see that consensus is building fast, suggesting that for all of us in midlife, a slow aggregation of proteins begin to block communication between the cells, resulting in mild forgetfulness. That's annoying, but it isn't pathological. In some people, for reasons that

I'll go into later, these same tiny proteins get out of control, triggering the development of dense plaques and tangles that surround neurons and eventually strangle them. Today, scientists are working hard to develop a test that will show—at the earliest possible moment—who is taking the wrong fork in the road.

That the seeds were already flourishing in some of us made for a grim prospect, but David Bennett, the director of the Alzheimer's Disease Center at Rush University Medical Center in Chicago, refused to look at it that way. "What's grim," he said, "is to call it 'normal aging,' to tuck your tail between your legs and refuse to put up a fight, both individually and on the political front." For the first time in history, he explained, the federal government has reduced the dollars they'll spend on Alzheimer's research. If you live to the age of fifty, there's an excellent chance that you'll make it into your late eighties.

"If you survive that long, your lifetime risk of developing Alzheimer's is very high," Bennett said. "If you don't want to end your life this way, you need to let Washington know about it. How fast we can get this disease under control depends largely on how much money we can throw at it. One primary prevention trial costs more than $30 million and takes five to ten years. So write to your representative in Congress and tell them you want a treatment by the time you're seventy."

Here's what is clear: No matter how innocent or malevolent your proteins are, how you treat your brain and the rest of your body in middle age will definitely make a difference. In response to considerable pressure from those of us in midlife, scientists have now turned their headlights on cognitive aging. A clear picture has emerged: Except for a very few individuals, who carry a specific genetic mutation, Alzheimer's is not the inevitability that we once imagined. Recent studies demonstrate that midlife is the time to act: to consider your diet, control your weight and blood sugar, amend your sleeping habits, increase your aerobic fitness, attend to your stress level and—most crucially—assure that your brain gets the right kind of exercise. These practices will go a long way toward making sure *you* take the right fork in the road, reaching old age with the bulk of your marbles intact.

2

GLITCHES, GAPS AND GAFFES

· · ·

The Memory-Hungry Crowd Speaks Candidly

About Screwing Up

Occasionally, I encounter someone who, despite the chronological onset of middle age, proudly claims to possess a memory like a steel trap. As the embarrassed owner of the cognitive equivalent of a kitchen sieve, I listen with interest. "Eureka, I've found one," I say to myself, and the hairs on my arms stand on end. I want to believe that such people exist.

Within a few minutes, I am almost always disappointed. One woman, a senior executive managing a workforce of four hundred, all of whom she claimed to know by name, had bent my ear at lunch, assuring me that her memory was unscathed. In fact, she confided, it was better than ever. I mentioned that I'd just had a conversation with Brian, a close friend of her husband's. "Brian?" she asked, surprised. "How do you know him?" To remind her that I'd sat next to him at a dinner party *at her house* seemed too cruel. In another disappointment, the father of one of my son's friends, a crackerjack trader on the stock exchange, promised me that his memory was still tops. It had to be, he explained. All day long, he kept track of puts and calls in his head. Could I imagine the disaster that would ensue if he *forgot*? I'd barely made note of that when he phoned back. He'd just realized that he couldn't drive the kids over to our house, as we'd planned. That morning, he'd taken his car to the shop.

People who boasted about their memories were usually kidding themselves. But I came across one notable exception—my friend Chloe, who writes books for young teenagers. She's well into her seventies now, and one could forgive her the occasional lapse. But she never forgets anything—not even the details of a conversation we had two decades ago, when apparently I told her I'd never consider coloring my hair. Recently, her son, now in his forties, phoned to ask her if she knew where he'd find his baptismal certificate. She swiveled in her desk chair and opened the second drawer of the filing cabinet. "I had it in my hand before he could finish explaining why he needed it," she said.

"How do you do it?" I asked her. "I never use electronic calendars, reminders, Palm Pilots or anything else," she explained. "I have a five-by-seven spiral-bound notebook and an ordinary desk calendar. All kinds of things get jotted down with the date during phone conversations—what an editor said, trip plans, holiday menus for the family, the name of the guy who does garden work—it's all there, but I depend on my memory of associated events to retrieve it. For instance, I think to myself, I had that discussion shortly before I had dinner with so-and-so, and then I can find the notes. Invariably, the friend who gave me the name of the gardener calls to ask me if I still have it, and I know where to look for the number."

Chloe, it should go without saying, is the exception. The rest of us are human.

"My memory is like a minefield," declared Evelyn, the songwriter. "Every once in a while, out of the blue, and for no apparent reason, I seem to stumble into an area that blows up in my face. The name of someone I know well is a complete mystery to me, or I forget the very thing I just swore to my husband I'd do. I'm always relieved when someone else slips up in my presence. It helps me accept the fact that I'm fallible, like everybody else."

AT WORK AND AT HOME

When I asked people whether they were more concerned about memory lapses at work or at home, most reported that there were un-limited opportunities for foul-ups in both places, not to mention those that emerged in the work-home transition, where some real doozies occur. In general, they agreed that forgetfulness at work scared them more. "After all," said Andrea, a psychologist, "my family can't fire me for being forgetful. My patients definitely will." Many reported moments during meetings and presentations when their ideas slipped away and they fervently desired to fall through a hole in the floor.

Fran, the marketing director at a bank, recalled a corporate meeting where she forgot three out of the six points she intended to present. "It made no sense," she said. "I'd rehearsed in the car. I'd ticked them off on my fingers. I had them down cold. And then they were gone." For her, the experience was deeply unsettling. "It never occurred to me that this could happen. I doubt I'll ever go into a meeting feel-ing relaxed and secure again," she said. At least she hadn't told the same person the identical thing, several times over. Marcy, a teacher, could lay claim to that error. "Repeating yourself, without the slight-est clue that you're doing it, is so tedious and middle-aged," she said. "I hate it."

Christine, for many years a human rights advocate, found at around fifty-five she could no longer handle her caseload. "I realized that I was unable to remember things and people I knew I should remem-ber," she told me. "When this happened several times, I knew it was affecting my ability to do my job. I didn't tell anyone why I left, but that was the reason." She took up a new, less memory-intensive pro-fession: innkeeping. There's still a lot to keep track of, including the names of a constantly changing parade of guests. "But now it's more about clean sheets and a good breakfast," she conceded, "rather than a matter of life and death."

Roger knew something about that. Now an attorney in private practice, he'd worked in southern California as an air-traffic control specialist for nearly three decades. "I was a cowboy, a real hotshot, for many years," he told me over breakfast, "but as I entered my forties, I could feel my brain changing. The ATC's job requires that you have ample working memory as well as long-term memory. You have to be fast enough and precise enough to continually make the right decision. You can't be sitting there asking yourself, 'Will I have enough memory to get me through the next rush of airplanes?' When you work in a dynamic safety profession, forgetting one thing can be lethal."

Each plane has its own call sign, Roger explained, and a single ATC can be in charge of a long string of jets, all attempting to land within minutes of each other at LAX. "The wrong call comes out of your mouth, or no call comes to mind," he said, "and you may or may not have time to reacquire the necessary information. That's very different from forgetting a phone number or the name of the person to whom you were just introduced."

As Roger's memory and attention started to dwindle, he found that even a short vacation threw him for a loop. "I'd come back, and damn, I'd need to refresh my memory. Trivial bits that can become critical if the right situation arises were not available to me." Slowly, he ramped down, leaving the unbearably stressful atmosphere of LAX's control tower for smaller fields. The all-but-mandatory retirement age for air-traffic controllers is fifty-six, but Roger ducked out nearly a decade earlier. "I had enough set by so that I could move on," he said. You wouldn't think that going to law school would work out for someone who was experiencing a memory deficit, but compared to life in the control tower, studying law was relaxing. "Next to the average Joe, my mind is pretty good," he remarked. "But there came a point where it wasn't good enough to stake thousands of lives on it every day."

For people who are trying to rejoin the workforce after years at home or hoping to change careers, the learning curve could seem impossibly steep. Claire, who received her Ph.D. in molecular biology twenty-five years ago, decided last year to leave her job in genetic engineering to take a position as a high school science teacher. Studying for the licensing exam, which recent college graduates pass with ease, was far more difficult than she'd anticipated. "I'm confident that I know what there is to know about high school molecular biology and genetics," she sighed. "But I haven't reviewed general science since early in college, and I don't seem to have enough memory available to hang on to all that information. Teaching high school has been a dream of mine for a long time, and it makes me crazy to think that my middle-aged brain may not allow me to pursue it."

Inevitably, forgetfulness plagues us at the most inconvenient and embarrassing moments. Lisbeth, who handles workers' compensation claims for the state of California, left her ATM card in the cash machine—three times. Carrie, a bookkeeper, stood outside the front door of a long-time client's office, desperately trying to remember the security code she'd punched in for a decade. "How could I call upstairs and ask for the number?" she asked. "How would that look?"

Forgetting what you intended to say in a meeting or finding it impossible to hang on to information is frustrating, but in terms of making you wonder if you're losing your marbles nothing compares to forgetting to do something you promised to do for someone else. Suddenly, your perception of yourself as a reliable, caring individual is called on the carpet. When my buddy Jerry, with whom I'd exchanged no fewer than nine e-mails in the previous week, nevertheless forgot and stood me up for breakfast, I teased him about it on the phone, and then ate my granola and drank my coffee alone, assuming that we'd reschedule for another day. He, on the other hand, was beside himself, spouting a string of self-flagellating four-letter words, convinced that his overtaxed middle-aged brain cells were perishing in large numbers. This terrible thing had happened, he explained, because he'd left his office the night before without taking the paper schedule he'd conscientiously printed out. It was still lying there in the printer tray. Out of sight, he said, was definitely out of mind.

It's horrible to stand up a friend (selfish!) or a colleague (flaky!), but consider what happened to Sean, who left fifty people standing around waiting for a presentation he'd carefully entered into his calendar—on the wrong day. "I was just getting home from work, opening the garage door," he said, "when my cell phone rang and this really pissed-off sounding woman hissed, 'Where are you?' I thought it was a crank call, but it wasn't. I'd messed up really bad."

In a similar vein, Peggy reported that a few weeks earlier, a friend who knew she made a regular northbound commute called to ask for a lift, so he could reclaim his car from the mechanic's. She wanted to run a five-minute errand, she told him, and would fetch him in about twenty minutes. It wasn't until she'd driven for an hour, well past the exit she'd have taken to deliver him to his vehicle, that she realized she'd forgotten to pick him up. "He was livid, and I felt like crawling into a hole and dying," she said. "He is truly one of the most easygoing people I know, but apparently, this was the last straw. Having him lose his temper with me only made the experience more searingly awful." John, a cardiologist, executed what must be the ultimate act of forgetfulness: He became so engrossed in the work he was doing on the computer that he failed to attend his aunt's funeral.

Until you forget something that has to do with a child (and there's hardly a parent who hasn't), you don't know what it feels like to be bathed in shame. When Marcy's daughter was in eighth grade, the girl took a day trip on a ski bus with some classmates, secure in the knowledge that her mother would collect her at 11:00 P.M. from the school's parking lot. "I wasn't there," Marcy admitted. "I was actually engrossed in a project at my desk, and I forgot about her completely. The director of the program had to drive her home, and I was very embarrassed."

The worst part is the rising sense that something is wrong. It comes upon you like flood waters: only seconds elapse between the time you notice that the basement floor is wet and the moment that you are up to your neck in remorse. There's nothing quite like it for killing your self-confidence and engendering free-floating anxiety in your children, especially if on an early-release Wednesday you've left them standing outside their school in pounding, horizontal rain, hail the size of golf balls and high winds, while you sit through a long meeting. The only known equivalent to failing to pick up a kid is failing to show up at a school performance. "I forgot which day my son was doing a poetry reading," mourned Georgia. "I still think of him up there in front of the classroom with fellow students, teachers and parents, with his mother and father nowhere to be seen, and it makes me sad. The day it happened, a few of the other mothers called, surprised I hadn't been there."

Forgetting how things work is nowhere near as psychologically devastating as forgetting your obligation to someone, but it's very annoying. People who successfully assembled thousand-part Lego sets in early parenthood learn in midlife that they can no longer follow directions. They get tangled up and lost, fitting together the pieces of Ikea dressers in the wrong order. Then they spend hours trying to take them apart again. Any kind of directions can pose a problem: Cooking complicated recipes, once a pleasant diversion for many, becomes a little too challenging when you forget what you're supposed to do next after each and every step.

In an essay in the *Atlantic Monthly*, "If Memory Doesn't Serve," Ian Frazier summed it up: "My son, who is eleven, has a memory like wet cement. Occurrences leave impressions on it and are there to stay—clear, manifest, close at hand. Like apparently all children today, he has an effortless affinity with gadgetry that exhausts me just to look at it. I call him when I want some advanced appliance turned off or on. Even more useful is his ability to replay data he observed. Ask him what we were talking about before we started talking about what we are talking about now, and he knows." Preadolescent children, handy as they are, are not always available when you need them. "I have taught myself the steps involved in creating a mail-merge in Microsoft Word at least four times," Sarah, a fund-raiser, told me. "And then I don't do it for a few months, and I have to start again, from scratch."

Forgetting how to perform a complex procedure over time is understandable. But losing track of something simple, like what you've just read, is enough to make you snap your crackers. This can occur on a microscale: You make it to the paragraph's end and find that you don't have a clue about what came before. Or it can occur on a macro level, when, for instance, you go out and buy a book you already own or have previously read. "That happens to me far too often," explained Jane, who has three preadolescent children. "Magazines, novels, you name it. My record is three times. Apparently, I'm reading with about a quarter of my brain. If that." Erica, who writes speeches for the CEO of a Fortune 500 company, admitted that she'd praised the novel *Beaches* to her husband, only to learn that the couple had seen the movie together. Her mate was able to recount the plot in excruciating detail, though during her reading it hadn't struck her as remotely familiar.

In an intimate relationship, marital or otherwise, forgetfulness can make you feel like you've been officially appointed the brunt of all jokes. In a courtship you're expected to remember, in substantial detail, the majority of things you've done together. Adam, a journalist in his midforties, fell in love with a woman who wasn't quite thirty. "In retelling the story of our courtship to friends," he remarked, "I seemed confused about certain details my fiancée remembered with clarity." At least he wasn't still out there, experiencing the joys of computer dating, where keeping track of whom you've met can be challenging. "A couple of nights back, I phoned a woman and asked her for a first date," said Rudy, who'd been out with a couple of dozen people in the last year. "She told me we'd had coffee two weeks earlier. From her tone of voice, which was a little chilly, I gathered that it had not been a success."

"I just broke up with a man who has the worst memory," said Katie, who works in sales for a printing company. "Last summer, he took me to Oliveto's for lunch, and we had a horrible fight. Six months later, we made up. For our reunion, he said we were going to try a wonderful new place, but then he took me straight back to the scene of the crime."

Wisely, she called a cab. If she'd married him, I'm sure she would have found herself on sweep-up duty, in charge of remembering just about everything. The contribution of the person who manages all the details is rarely recognized—until it becomes evident that with age he or she is slipping. Laura's absentminded musician husband gratefully put her in charge of the calendar as soon as they were married. That worked well enough for twenty years, until she turned fifty. "To have me slip up now is really blowing many of our sacrosanct beliefs about who we are as a couple," she said.

The genders, I've found, have very different attitudes toward forgetfulness. Women usually adopt the customary mea culpa stance; if they've neglected to remind a teenage child of a standing appointment, well, we know whose fault *that* is. They're quick to blame menopause for anything from missing keys to a car they can't find in the shopping mall parking lot, although studies show that estrogen—or its absence—affects only verbal memory. Men have no such biological crutch, so they lean on the theory of selective memory. Within earshot of their wives, many told me how they unfailingly remembered what was important to them, and forgot everything else. "I suppose your selective memory was to blame last Saturday, when you forgot to pick up Sammy from soccer," Louise said, rolling her eyes. "And our last anniversary, which you remembered at the eleventh hour? Was that selective memory, too?" I found that men are often unaware of their sturdy automatic reminder systems, in the form of wives and assistants. "I have a secretary and technology to keep me on track at work, so I am unlikely to forget anything," the male editor of a business magazine told me. "As the boss, I delegate a lot. So, in a curious way, it's other peoples' responsibility to remind me of things." The true state of affairs is often not obvious until the wife takes a two-week trip to Vietnam with her best girlfriend or the assistant departs for maternity leave. Then, the forgetting begins.

When it's time to find something—a restaurant or a missing notebook—that's when it's evident that male and female brains are not exactly the same. There are good evolutionary reasons behind a woman's ability to give you the precise coordinates of a dusty can of garbanzo beans in the back of the pantry, and the old but true saw about men refusing to stop to ask for directions. Because males emerged as hunters, without the benefit of gas stations where they could ask directions, they developed internal global positioning systems. Millions of years later, they continue to navigate by *feeling* their way to their destinations. Learning that there's a Nordstrom's at the second stoplight is of no particular help. As gatherers with small children who were likely to be snatched, women's brains developed differently. They couldn't travel far, so they learned to track down food sources — nuts, berries and roots — that were embedded in complex arrays of vegetation, much of which was poisonous. And that may well explain why a woman can tell you that your missing green sock is on the floor between the nightstand and the bed, and a man can't track down the scissors that have resided in the same kitchen drawer for eleven years.

NO MARGIN FOR ERROR

Many people told me how much they hated the time they wasted while they retraced their steps, trying to clean up the messes they'd made. "Do you know how often I refer to an attachment in an e-mail, and then forget to send the attachment?" asked Bart, a graphic artist. "More often, I think, than I actually send it." He'd be happy to know that two scientists at the University of Pennsylvania are developing software that scans e-mails for characteristics that suggest that something ought to be attached. If you try to send that sucker off without adding your file, you'll get a message. So far, the software is about 85 percent accurate, which certainly represents an improvement on Bart's current record.

Our lapses might be more tolerable if our schedules weren't packed to the hilt. As it stands, there's no margin for error. Russell, a practicing physician and busy researcher, remarked that on a long return flight from a business trip, he abandoned his prescription reading glasses on the plane. "I must have put them in the seatback pocket and forgotten them," he said. "That it was going to cost money to replace them was bad enough, but the fact that there wasn't a single unaccounted-for minute in the next two weeks made it worse. I might as well have had to climb Mount Everest."

At least he didn't have to explain it to his wife. Pat, who practices alternative medicine, lost track of where she hid the earrings her husband gave her on the occasion of their twentieth anniversary, which made it impossible for her to wear them to dinner at Spago on their twenty-first. "I tore the house apart looking," she said. "I stayed up at night while Rick slept and went through the closet. When I couldn't find them, I thought I'd just call the insurance company and replace them, and he'd never have to know. It turned out that I needed the receipt, so I had to confess. I started dramatically: 'Honey, there's something I need to tell you.' When he figured out that I was talking about lost earrings, he was relieved. He said, 'Oh, thank God. I thought you were leaving me.'"

Forgetfulness, in the form of lost belongings and missed appointments, can get expensive, which makes it all the more irritating. Carly, who works for a museum, said that she'd missed—and paid for—a few appointments with the hairdresser, each of which she'd carefully scheduled six weeks in advance. "I keep a calendar, meticulously, but a lot of the time I forget to look at it," she said. "I'm not even good at remembering regularly scheduled meetings. On a pretty regular basis I forget and schedule another meeting on top of the one I have every Tuesday morning. The situation is not yet hopeless, but it can be pretty frustrating."

What I hate most, I think, are the errors that arise out of what I refer to as negative space. The term encompasses everything for which there is not a single helpful cue, no list or calendar item on hand that might assist. I got lost in negative space last summer, after I wrote the final check in my checkbook and replaced it with a fresh packet I took from a box in my lower desk drawer. I paid several large bills, posting them so that they would arrive safely by their due dates. Three days later, I received a call from the bank, telling me that the checks were written on an account that had been closed for four years. Frankly, I found this unbelievable. I had no recollection of ever having, or closing, such an account.

"Did you look at the account number printed on the bottom of check?" the patient assistant bank manager inquired. When I compared it to the number that belonged to my current account, I could see that we were indeed talking apples and oranges. Every check I'd written, she regretted to tell me, including the one I'd sent to pay the first invoice from my new MasterCard account, the bank would return with "account closed" stamped across it in red. There was nothing I could do to remedy the situation. As far as the credit card company was concerned, I was guilty of check kiting. In addition to being furious at myself, I felt helpless and stupid. Eventually, I got a nice, middle-aged lady on the phone and explained the situation in detail. It could have happened to anyone, she agreed—and kindly restored my account to working order.

3

FRONTAL-LOBE OVERLOAD

· · ·

"Too Much Information" Is Just One of

the Reasons You Feel Like You're Drowning

My mind was behaving like a car radio on a lonesome road, drift-ing from station to station without ever locking in on a signal. While I tried to recall the order of San Francisco's hilly streets—was it Buchanan, Webster and Laguna?—I glanced quickly at my Palm Pilot, checking yet again for the address of the dermatologist's office. In a split second, I forgot it.

As usual, I was thinking about too many things—Osama, freshly alarming in that morning's video; an upcoming deadline for a maga-zine article; and whether I had enough time, if I stayed up all night, to make costumes for the school play. Okay, I admit it: I'd been on the cell phone, too. Around the time the motorist in front of me cut me off (or did I just fail to notice his blinker?), I realized I'd passed my destination by some blocks, requiring a spatially challenging series of right-hand turns down one-way streets and alleys.

couldn't I multitask well enough to encode a street name and
digits? Why was I so distracted? My absentmindedness shocked
me. Newly minted ideas slipped away before I could summon com-
patible or contradictory notions and introduce them to each other.
Intentions that were perfectly evident to me while I was getting
dressed—"take two reams of printer paper to the office"—popped
like evanescent bubbles before I made it downstairs to the supply cabinet in the garage. Repeatedly, I was shocked by the total erasure of
the obligation. Not until I hit the print button on my keyboard and
heard the empty paper tray groan in protest did I develop the faintest
recollection of my plan.

The problem, it seemed, lay somewhere behind my forehead, in
the region of the brain called the prefrontal cortex. More specifically,
my frontal lobes were acting their age. The frontal lobes guide the
organization and prioritization of information and ideas, decision
making and planning, time management and various other cognitively
demanding, uniquely human tasks.

To understand what was going on, I had to begin at a cellular level.
Under the patient guidance of a researcher at MIT, I studied a neuron
through an electron microscope. The diamond-shaped cell body
vaguely resembled a starfish, with multiple tentacles. Each tentacle
sprouted branches called dendrites, festooned with synapses as lush
and thick as the foliage of a California oak. One tentacle, the axon,
was noticeably longer than the others. This spindly extremity, decked
out in a string of sausage-shaped beads of lipid fat called the myelin
sheath, transmits signals to the dendrites of other neurons. The frontal
lobes are packed with long, stringy axons which link one region of the
brain with another. When myelin starts to decay, axons don't work
quite as well. Instead of traveling the superhighways, information
takes some inconvenient detours. The results are predictable: Data
you really need, right this second, shows up in its own sweet time.

Under the electron microscope, I examined the synapse, a complicated little stub at the very end of the axon. The synapse transmits
electrochemical signals, impulses that race down the cell body from
dendrite to axon, before leaping into a Pac-Man style gap. Neurotrans-

mitters, released into the gap, are sucked up by other cells' hungry dendrites, thus transferring impulses from one cell to another. The number of receptors and the availability of neurotransmitters largely determine how fast and accurately messages will travel.

The frontal lobes provide us with working memory, the faculty that allows us to store and manipulate information over short periods of time until it is transferred into long-term memory. As species go, we're not robustly endowed with working memory—even chimps have more. Scientists suspect that the earliest *Homo sapiens* traded off a chunk of working memory to the development of language, a worthwhile swap as long as you can remember what it was that you intended to say. When working memory is impaired, it becomes difficult to remember the thread of an argument, to make a point or, for that matter, to recall what you read three sentences earlier. Instead of flowing freely, your thoughts become disjointed. As the late Yale neuroscientist Patricia Goldman-Rakic observed, working memory is "the mental glue that links a thought through time from its beginning to its end."

When the frontal lobes are in top form, they're adept at figuring out what's important for the job at hand and what's irrelevant blather. A sort of neural bouncer automatically evicts unnecessary information. Some time in middle age, that bouncer takes a permanent coffee break. Instead of thinking about the report that's due, you find yourself considering what to cook for dinner. For many people, preoccupation has become a way of life. "I do not live in the present," said Louise, the mother of two elementary school children. "I am always three or four steps ahead of where I actually am. My mind is never completely processing what is happening to me while it is happening." Indeed, any emotional distraction can tie up your brain's switchboard, leaving you preoccupied and self-absorbed, even when you know you shouldn't be. Try to do something "important" and you're likely to get a busy signal.

Whether it is environmental—a barking dog or an irritating neighbor—or psychological—intrusive thoughts about the fight you had with your wife—the midlife brain is easily confounded by what neuroscientist Denise Park calls "background noise." In one of her investigations, she tested two groups, one middle-aged and the other composed of older seniors, on an everyday memory task—remembering to take medication at 10:00 A.M. To her surprise, the older group's performance far surpassed that of her middle-aged subjects. Park postulated that for older individuals, swallowing that pill became a significant feature of their morning's schedule. Midlifers, whose schedules are typically irregular, were juggling so many competing tasks in working memory that pill taking fell by the wayside.

COULD IT BE ADHD?

Who can blame us for wanting to find a name for feeling so scatter-brained? During our interviews, dozens of people confided in me that they knew exactly what was wrong with them: They'd developed adult ADHD. I'd wondered about it myself, so I phoned psychiatrist and author Edward M. Hallowell, who has diagnosed attention deficit disorders in his private practice in Sudbury, Massachusetts, since 1981. When he invited me to come to see him, I jumped at the chance. I was sure he could tell me what had caused my attention to fracture into a million tiny pieces.

I barely stifled my laughter when I saw his office. There were small, medium-size and large piles of paper stacked on the floor, like so many budding stalagmites, one of the top indicators that ADHD is in the house. Hallowell resembled a young Ted Kennedy, bright white hair framing a ruddy, full face that nearly matched his candy-striped shirt. He asked me diagnostic questions: What had I been like as a child? Had I been able to sit still? To concentrate? I was a bookworm, I told him, the kind of kid who sneaks a flashlight under the covers, even though she's already been reading for hours. Stick me in a ballet class or a game with teams and lots of rules, and it got ugly. It was hard for me to focus, to learn the steps, to get with the program. In school, I was fine—those rules, I knew by heart. He wanted to know about my work habits as an adult. Did I procrastinate? Did I have trouble getting started, or for that matter, completing one assignment before embarking on another? I did not, I told him. In fact, I was the opposite—once I was engaged, I was inclined to hyperfocus. Like a greyhound after a rabbit, I could not be made to change my course.

If I found myself in a relaxing setting, Hallowell inquired—a lovely hotel room, or in a lawn chair by a peaceful lake—how would I feel? Did I crave excitement? Was I soon off to book a parasailing experience or a jet ski—or was I content to simply sit and read? The latter, I assured him. Give me a lawn chair, a book and a sufficient amount of chef's salad and lemonade and I'd stay put, gratefully, for a week.

After some further probing into other aspects of my neurological function— How was my balance? (Terrible) Could I stand on one foot? (Never, to my yoga teacher's disgust)—he told me that my symptoms didn't stack up as ADHD. Some other, unspecified malaise had apparently affected my frontal lobes. He could not say whether or not there was pathology involved. At the least, he guessed I had a bad case of a syndrome so common among middle-aged people he'd given it a name. He called it ADT—attention deficit trait. As opposed to ADHD, which goes with you wherever you wander, ADT is an environmentally induced frontal-lobe shutdown.

When the demands are unceasing, Hallowell observed, "when you are confronted with the sixth decision after the fifth interruption in the midst of a search for the ninth missing piece of information on the day that the third deal has collapsed and the twelfth impossible request has blipped unbidden across your computer screen," your brain rebels against excessive stimuli. "It's purely a response to the hyperkinetic environment in which we live," he explained, "emerging as a survival mechanism, our answer to society's demand to move faster and faster."

MANAGING THE ONSLAUGHT OF INFORMATION

Under the best of circumstances, middle-aged frontal lobes have a hard time keeping pace. Drop them smack in the middle of a technological revolution, and you've got a recipe for trouble. Over millions of years, the human brain has sensibly evolved to attend to events that might threaten our survival. It was not designed to deal with an unstoppable deluge of data—raw, unfiltered, out of context and without an obvious hierarchy. Our frontal lobes are ill equipped to handle the onslaught, which leaves us feeling bombarded, overwhelmed and out of control. In one of its theatrical productions, the performers known as the Blue Man Group refer to "Info-Biological Inadequacy Syndrome," a form of anxiety, observes author David Shenk in his book, *Data Smog*, "brought on when a person wishes he could absorb information at a rate somewhat faster than the level that was hard-wired into the human DNA back in the Paleolithic era."

When the frontal lobes overload, our ability to think at higher levels disappears. In response, we erect a sturdy perceptual filter, a sort of diaphanous mesh, and begin to screen out a lot of things, including some revealed later to have merited closer attention. We stop processing the meaning of information and become robotic data suckers. Shenk notes that the relentless bombardment of the frontal lobes causes "paralysis by analysis." It's hard to arrive at a simple conclusion—there are just too many factors to consider. For many situations, we lack an appropriate frame of reference. We've become specialists, big kahunas in our own little fiefdoms. We wind up ignoring most of what is taking place around us, in a way that makes us feel spacily unobservant.

In an effort to protect ourselves, we become very concrete, inclined to eliminate all shades of gray from our reasoning and perspective. It becomes impossible to see how the pieces of the jigsaw puzzle fit together. "Metaphorically speaking, we plug up our ears, pinch our nose, cover our eyes with dark sunglasses and step into a body suit lined with protective padding," observes Shenk.

It's not the first time this has happened. Whenever we invent technology that allows us to mess with the limitations of time and space, people become distracted and forgetful. In less than a decade, between 1869 and 1876, the American transcontinental railroad was completed, Alexander Graham Bell invented the telephone and Thomas Edison greatly improved the existing lightbulb. Life changed dramatically, and people began to fall ill, developing a range of speed-and-time-related ailments, including "railway neurosis" and "elevator sickness." Most common was the catch-all diagnosis of "neurasthenia," which, observes Michelle Stacey in her book, *The Fasting Girl*, arose from "generalized anxiety, a sense of dread or worry, often brought on by an overload of demands on our abilities and time, or by an underlying apprehension of our capacity for self-destruction." One of the main symptoms of neurasthenia was a pathological deficit in attention that caused the patient to live life in a perpetual state of distraction.

The ambivalence we feel about managing the new technology and the reams of information that invariably accompany it has been a long time in the making. In 1945, while he was director of the wartime Office of Scientific Research and Development, Vannevar Bush struggled with the problem of information overload. Inspired by the recent invention of a new recording substrate, microfilm, he proposed a solution. In July of that year, he published an eight-page article in the *Atlantic Monthly* entitled "As We May Think." He laid out the future of information technology in striking detail, notes David Shenk. "Bush outlined the concepts of microfiches, modems, fax machines, personal computers, hard drives, voice-operated word processors and, most important, hypermedia. He imagined the future work desk—a memex, he called it—as a microlibrary filled with all the video and text that one person could accumulate in a lifetime, designed with the ability to retrieve relevant information instantaneously and project it onto a built-in display terminal."

Unfortunately, Bush was fixated on microfilm, a medium that anyone who reeled endlessly through it in the seventies and eighties can tell you lends itself more to frustration than speed or interactivity. When Bush died in 1974, the memex was still a fanciful notion. His *Atlantic Monthly* article found its way into the hands of a sufficient number of computer engineers, most of whom were laboring to program room-size computing devices. Bush never knew that his plan—making it possible for you or me to store nearly everything about a life—would come to fruition.

With this most recent explosion of technology (recall that fifteen years ago, only the most sophisticated computer buffs were online), we've experienced a backlash similar to the one that occurred in Thomas Edison's time. In his book, *In Praise of Slowness*, Carl Honoré captured the essence of our struggle: "In *Don Quixote*, Cervantes noted that '*Que no son todos los tiempos unos*'—not all times are the same. In a 24/7 world, however, all time is the same: we pay bills on Saturday, shop on Sunday, take the laptop to bed, work through the night, tuck into all-day breakfasts. We mock the seasons by eating imported strawberries in the middle of winter and hot cross buns, once an Easter treat, all year round. With cell phones, BlackBerrys, pagers and the Internet, everyone and everything is now permanently available."

"The world has become too immediate," asserted Lily, an office manager. "At one point, I had four voice-mail boxes, four phone numbers and three e-mail addresses I was responsible for checking. There's an overload of stuff, and although most of it isn't important, it still has to be looked at and disposed of. All those expressions we grew up with—'one thing at a time' and 'first things first'—have become archaic. As far as I can tell, there is no longer any such thing as a 'first thing.'"

We are in shock, caught between the world in which we grew to adulthood, one that ran on conventional chronology, and the one we live in now, which leaps over all boundaries. Robert Archibald, a historian, stated it well: "Change is an immutable law. But if change is too rapid in the world around us, we are bewildered, imprisoned in the present, disconnected from those around us and making do with relationships that are fragile, unmoored and unconfirmed."

People react to the pressure in different ways. Some become control freaks, fighting hard to manage every shred of information that comes their way. Others throw up their hands and let the wave overtake them. "I was dead tired," one correspondent told me, "because I'd just returned from a business trip in Europe, but the limousine service that always picks me up didn't show. When I phoned, the driver said that he'd forgotten me because my order had disappeared under a pile of papers on his desk. I wasn't happy. 'Well, I'm only human,' the driver told me, when I asked if it would happen again. I didn't feel very sympathetic."

To be fractured has become a societal expectation. To refuse to be so—no e-mail, no cell phone, no voice mail—is not only Luddite, but oddly selfish. If we had slipped into middle age in a calmer era—perhaps 1953, when the really big deal for our parents was the half-dozen TV channels from which you were free to choose—we might not notice the decline of our frontal lobes. As it stands, we've arrived smack in the middle of a technological revolution that has left us gasping for air and struggling to stay afloat. Unless you are willing to make it your business to be mentally ubiquitous and reachable except when you are unconscious, you have the sense that you are falling behind. It is futile, shortsighted and probably hypocritical to rail against our device-driven existence. I would not argue for a second that we'd be better off without the ability to find out almost anything at any time. Personally, I develop an itchy mouse finger when I have the need to know and no immediate way to find out. Take me away from the information nipple for any length of time and I develop data starvation. Any day, I'm expecting to get what one man described as "the Google chip, the silicon implant that plugs all of Google directly into our brains."

In an essay in the *New York Times*, Adam Bryant wrote a touching farewell letter to his BlackBerry, a company-issued perk he'd relinquished when he left his job. He'd assumed that his BlackBerry made him more productive, but in its absence, he'd learned that it was "a black hole of attention," sucking hours from his days and haunting his nights. "I thought you were under my thumbs," he wrote, "but I was under yours."

When Jane's hybrid phone, e-mail and calendaring device suddenly died, taking valuable data with it, she was furious at the equipment and even angrier at herself because she hadn't backed it up in a month or two. "I felt that I had been deceived," she said. "I had trusted the thing and it let me down." Within a few days, she realized that her life was calmer. "Now I can do exactly one thing at a time," she remarked with satisfaction. "When I had it, I felt compelled to check it whenever I had a few minutes, to plan things or to replan things that had already been planned."

Her three children and her husband are annoyed with her. So are her friends. Even her therapist wants to know when she is going to get a replacement. "It's a bit of a fuck you," she said, obviously enjoying her moment of rebellion, "to be unreachable in this day and age."

Some suspect that these impossible-to-live-without conveniences may be the catalysts for our cognitive problems. "We are too dependent on technology as a tool of storage," mused Victor, an economist. "Without exercising the brain by having to dig for information, over time we may lose some important abilities." If the results of a recent study by researchers at the Hokkaido University School of Medicine are accurate, the decline is already evident in people in their twenties and thirties, who so compulsively finger their tiny keypads that they are called *oyayubizoku*, the "thumb tribe." According to neurobiology professor Toshiyuki Sawaguchi, about one in ten of the forty individuals his group studied had "lost the ability to remember new things, to pull out old data or to distinguish between important and unimportant information." The predominance of electronic organizers, speed dials, spell checkers and automobile GPS devices resulted in diminished use of the brain, making regions involved in learning and memory become flimsy and weak.

Even the things that are designed to help us are often too complicated or memory-intensive to be of use. "My telephone at work came with a one-hundred-page manual," said Victor. "Consumer electronic devices have a massive number of features, but access to these is neither intuitive nor standardized. Why can't all voice-mail systems use the *D* key for delete and the *S* key for save? As it is, I have six phone numbers, three voice mails and five e-mail accounts." When I asked Jeff Hawkins, the chief technology officer at Palm, why the buttons you punch for various services on the Treo, Palm's hybrid phone and organizer, could not be standardized to help out midlifers, he confided that people my age (which, as it happens, is also his age) and older are not really their market. The keypads are too small and the interfaces too complex and too infrequently tackled to allow anyone who is not a digital whiz to catch on. I own a Treo, I told him, and I've got the basic functions down. But I'll be damned if I can figure out how to make a note or jot down a telephone number in the address book while I'm in the middle of a call. My Verizon contract on the Treo is nearly up. I'm due for a new one, but I dread the transition.

A TOUGH HABIT TO BREAK

"The real challenge of modern life," observed Edward Hallowell, the psychiatrist, "is to be able to stop and think, to pause over one point long enough to extract what matters before moving on. Otherwise, the day becomes a blur in which no significant work gets done. . . . For the energy to get focused, a person must be able to put the brakes on incoming stimuli and outgoing impulses long enough to concoct a complex thought."

That's unfortunate, because an endless stream of interruptions has become the norm. Researchers at the University of California, Irvine attempted to quantify the number of distractions and interruptions that occur among IT workers in a medium-sized office. They predicted that something would interfere with concentration every fifteen minutes, but on average, interruptions occurred every three minutes, and only two-thirds of the interrupted work was resumed on the same day. Another study showed that interruptions take up over two hours of each working day, at an estimated cost to the U.S. economy of $588 billion annually. All these interruptions result in some terrible mistakes, observed one survey respondent. The ease with which he can copy people on an e-mail means that, inevitably, those errors go viral. The wrong date for the meeting is sent not to one person, but to twenty.

Even when you know what's going on, it's difficult to break the automatic habit of fracturing attention. We've grown so accustomed to overstimulation that operating within the parameters of human neurological function feels painfully slow. By multitasking, we can alleviate discomfort caused by our snail-like pace, but that relief is likely to be brief. As the frontal lobes' ability to cast off distracting information declines, our mistakes multiply alarmingly.

"It used to feel so good," wrote June, a tax attorney. "I could do at least three things at once, and do all of them well. A couple of years ago, things started breaking down. When I was trying to talk on the phone and read my e-mail at the same time, my sentences became incomprehensible. I couldn't fold the laundry and have a meaningful conversation with my daughter. At first, the breakdowns were disappointing, but then they became disastrous, resulting in mistakes, lost papers and confusion. You'd think I would have stopped. But I couldn't imagine a different strategy. When it works, you feel so competent and you get so much done. It was the only way I knew to be efficient."

Even much younger people, who grew up with their fingers on a computer keyboard, have trouble doing more than one thing at a time. Using neuroimaging, MIT psychologist Yuhong Jiang watched the working brains of college students as they tried to accomplish two relatively straightforward tasks simultaneously. After a half hour of practice, these young, highly accomplished subjects were still stressed by the effort of switching back and forth from identifying shapes to identifying colors and letters. Images from the brain scanner showed that between tasks, the frontal lobes were taking a snooze. They went blank, as if awaiting instructions.

Studies executed by David E. Meyer at the University of Michigan showed that, except for the most routine endeavors, it was more time-consuming and wearying for the brain to alternate between tasks than it would be if the same jobs were done one at a time. "If both tasks require strategic thought," noted Marcel Just, a psychology professor at Carnegie Mellon, "you're out of luck. The strategic control system in the brain is really hard to share. Every time you attempt it, it's the equivalent of clearing your desk, laying out all the new work, and then switching it back to the way it was before. It's not like you can sneak in another task in the background." There are exceptions, he acknowledged. Although it can be messy, you can eat and read at the same time. In theory, you should be able to stir a pot and watch television, although I've proved otherwise.

I let June, the tax attorney, in on what I'd learned. "I decided to back off and try to do just two things at a time," she reported. "But that didn't work either. Finally, I realized that I could stop trying so hard and things would get better. Now, instead of egging myself on to multitask, I say, 'One thing at a time, finish this before you start that, no, don't try to open the mail while you're on the phone, waiting for the computer to boot up.' It's all precious time, and I hate to waste it, but I remind myself that I'm screwing up much less."

It's so much the norm these days that it takes a certain amount of awareness to recognize that you're multitasking inefficiently. Hearing of June's success, I decided to consciously change my approach. The next time I had to locate a street address, I stopped trying to behave like a twenty-year-old. I put the phone down and left the yogurt container untouched on the passenger seat. I shoved Osama out of my mind, at least for the moment. Instead, I actually concentrated on the matter at hand, paying strict attention to such basics as street names and the tiny numbers that appear over San Francisco doorways. I arrived on time, calm, and even noted my space and floor number before I left the parking structure. "So simple," I thought as I pressed the correct elevator button and disembarked on the proper floor, as long as I remembered to act my age.

4

BLOCKING, BLANKING
AND BEGGING FOR MERCY
. . .
Why Words and Thoughts Flee Without Warning

As people completed and returned their surveys, I began to study and categorize their memory lapses, as if they were so many butterflies. There was Colliding Planets Syndrome, which occurs when you fail to grasp, until it is too late, that you've scheduled a child's orthodontist appointment in the suburbs for the same hour as a business meeting in the city. Temporal Geographic Complex causes you to show up at the wrong time, or in the wrong location, or both. What Am I Doing Here? Syndrome leaves you standing empty-handed in a doorway, trying to figure out what you've come for. Wrong Vessel Disorder results in placing the container of ice cream in the pantry, rather than in the freezer. The Damn It, It Was Just in My Hand Affliction leads to panicky moments spent searching for the check that moments earlier arrived in the mail. The Which Child, What Year?

Dilemma presents itself at an inconvenient moment, like when you are standing in the emergency room trying to decide if your teenager really needs a tetanus shot. Then, there is the mystifying Raised by Aliens Phenomenon, when you realize that you and your sister have substantially different recollections of your childhood.

EVERYBODY BLOCKS

All of these lapses are common in midlife, but there is one type of flub that is universal. Everyone describes the pain of the very public cognitive failure known as "blocking" (or "blanking"), when names will not come to mind and words dart in and out of consciousness, hiding in dark closets just when you need them. An eminent Alzheimer's researcher confessed that at every conference he attends he sees someone who was in his postdoctoral training program. "Maybe it was ten years back, or last year—I've had a couple of hundred at least," he said, "but invariably, this person is heading toward me. Of course he knows my name, and I have to do this little tricky thing with my glasses, sort of sliding them down my nose, so I can read his name tag without him knowing that I'm looking."

Blocking is by far the most common form of memory lapse. Kent, the general counsel for a credit card company, confides that he is able to recognize faces as familiar and identify people based on conceptual knowledge of who they are, but often blocks on the names of the people he's worked with every day for eighteen months. Henry, a magazine editor, observes that it isn't unusual for him to need to rise from his desk and check the nameplate on the outside wall of a staffer's cubicle before he can recall how to e-mail him. "When I say hello to someone by name who I see only a couple of times a year, I am wrong at least 50 percent of the time," he said. "It seems to be getting worse, so now I just nod." Gina, a book editor, said that she has blocked on the names of her own dinner guests, which made it difficult to introduce them to each other.

These kinds of things happen to me all the time. The sudden, unexpected absence of information confounds my ability to do things I do every day. For no reason at all, I can't remember the electrician's name, making it impossible to telephone him, although he's been at my house more times than I can count. I'm unable to recall the password that allows me to log on to my friend June's computer to check my e-mail, though I've asked her for it embarrassingly often. At the worst possible moment—in the middle of a business trip, with not a minute to spare—my ATM password goes AWOL. Words I know how to spell play games with me, and source memory—the ability to recall who said what to whom (and where)—goes on a brief vacation.

When that industrial-grade garage door slams shut in your mind, the only thing to do is to wait patiently until your brain is ready to do business. "What I experience," notes Karen, a grant writer, "is a momentary total blank. It happens most with abstract ideas, which don't have a lot of ready replacements. I'll be sitting there, trying to think of the word 'determination.' It's a word that would fit perfectly, except that I can't come up with it, nor can I produce a synonym that would allow me to look it up. I'm not getting a damned thing. The post office is closed."

Daniel Schacter, the renowned Harvard psychologist and expert on memory, explains that name and word blocking result from a weakened connection between visual and conceptual representations (things you know about a person or an object) and phonological representations (the sound of a word or a name). When such a connection hasn't been thoroughly made, or recently strengthened, the link becomes unreliable and you become susceptible to blocking.

In his landmark book, *The Seven Sins of Memory*, Schacter observes that the concept of blocking exists in fifty-one languages and that forty-five of those languages use phrases that include a mention of the tongue to describe a blocked item that felt like it was on the verge of recovery. The Cheyenne used an expression, *Navonotootse' a*, which translates as "I have lost it on my tongue." In Korean, it is *Hyeu kkedu-te-mam-do-da*, which in English means, "It's sparkling on the end of my tongue." However it is expressed, observes Schacter, the individual feels as though he is "in mild torment, something like on the brink of a sneeze." If he finds the word he is desperately trying to retrieve, his relief is considerable.

Studies show that in comparison with younger people, older adults produce more unspecific pronouns—words like "it"—than common or proper nouns, such as "the Deere tractor." An entire vocabulary has sprung up to compensate for TOTs (tip of the tongue lapses), notes William Safire in his *New York Times* column, "On Language." In addition to the ever descriptive "thing," there is "whichamahoozy, hoosydingy, watchamacallit, whodingy, doodad, gizmo, gadget, widget, doohicky, whoosit, thingamajig or even hootenanny." He left out my favorite, the all-encompassing "whosywhatsis."

To fend off a tip of the tongue incident, Schacter says, "you have to take a proactive stance. If you're going to a school meeting, re-lating to your kids, that's where you're likely to see people you feel you should know, but haven't seen recently or frequently. That's a recipe for a TOT name-blocking episode. It might take a heroic effort, but you should review the list of the names of people who are going to attend. Once you're there, and the blocking has occurred, it's too late."

In midlife and onward, resolving the TOT grows increasingly chal-lenging. In the split second between your query: "What do you call that sleek, dark purple vegetable?" and the response, "Eggplant," your aging brain, lacking the reliable neural bouncer I discussed earlier, de-livers quantities of unrequested information. Word-retrieval failures occur not because of the loss of relevant memories, but because irrele-vant ones are activated. Often, notes Schacter, "people can produce vir-tually everything they know about a person, or everything they know about a word, except its label." The brain volunteers words that begin with the same letter, items that are the same color, and my personal fa-vorite, words with the same number of syllables, all of which gum up the works. British psychologist James Reason named these persistent alternatives "ugly sisters," unwanted and intrusive words that force themselves upon you and prevent you from reaching a much-sought-after target. We tend to embrace the ugly sisters, remarks Schacter, because they provide us with the comforting feeling of being close to the target, and thus about to resolve the TOT. With age, both the persistent alternatives and the information available about the target word decrease, leaving you less sure than you were in your twenties about the word you sought.

Greg, a mortgage broker, told me that recently he'd blocked repeatedly on a word he knew perfectly well. "I live in a wooded environment with acres of weeds that need to be cleared regularly," he said. "There's a constant need to go out and pick Scotch broom. I have become obsessive in my desire to conquer the enemy. To my complete consternation I have found over the past few weeks that when my children ask where I am going, I can't produce the name of that weed. This symptom of my forgetfulness is both frustrating and perplexing, as I can find no rational explanation for forgetting a word that is so present in my life."

HOW WORDS MAKE IT OUT OF YOUR MOUTH

No matter what your age, the normal effort involved in turning a concept—egg-shaped, purple, smooth, shiny, funny green cap—into a word requires three levels of processing. At the first, or lexical level, you summon information about shape, color and utility, which generates a strong feeling of knowing—the sense that it is on the tip of your tongue. This millisecond-long search retrieves such data as the general appearance of the Greek restaurant where you enjoyed eating baba ghanoush, the color of a favored marking pen, the slick patent leather surface of a childhood raincoat. That accomplished, you step up to the next level, the lemma network, where you sift through your vocabulary, looking for something that matches, rejecting items that reflect some of the word's phonetic demands—egg salad? ice plant?—but not all. With increasing age, it takes more time to access these phonetic bits and pieces. If all goes well, at the lexeme level, you assemble the components. If you fail at one of these levels, you block—or worse, you allow some vaguely similar word to escape from your lips.

Whether you are hunting for a word, a name or your train of

thought, the moment of unblocking is explosive. "It's a brain avalanche," Victor, the economist, exclaimed. "You search and you search and then all the information floods in at once, usually a while after you've given up. The worst part is that when the dam breaks, you're bombarded with so many images and ideas that you become distracted and miss the next three things that happen."

The process breaks down in social situations, where name-blocking events most often occur. Anxiety kidnaps a chunk of your already limited working memory, leaving piddling amounts available for getting people's names straight and making introductions. "It happens to me all the time at parties where I'm supposed to meet new people," said June, the tax attorney. "I'm so busy worrying about what to say, and whether I'm being sufficiently interesting, that I can barely introduce myself, never mind manage the introduction of anyone else."

When anxiety surfaces, as it often does in these situations, it causes the individual to focus on the here and now, with a remarkable amount of degradation in memory. Time pressure is a major factor in blocking. It interferes both with storing and retrieving information, which explains why, when you're facing a major deadline or standing before a demanding audience, you find that you can't think straight. The time span from which knowledge can be easily retrieved (you met her at Martha's dinner party, four months ago) and used in a specific context (and now, you need to introduce her to Sarah, who's standing in front of you) shrinks as your stress level increases. Roman aristocrats avoided this situation by always traveling with a nomenclatur, an alert slave whose duty it was to supply his master with the names of acquaintances as they were encountered.

In the absence of such a companion, Barbara Wallraff, writing in the *Atlantic Monthly*, sought suggestions from her readers on how to describe the moment when you should introduce two people, but have blocked on their names. As names for the affliction, someone suggested "whomnesia." Others proposed "nomstruck," "nomenclature," and "mumbleduction." Managing the introduction by getting someone else to produce the name was called "introducking," and doing it without providing any names at all was called "introduping."

Comedienne and talk-show host Joan Rivers noted that she'd figured out two ways to deal with blocking. "Either I touch the person's chest and look like I'm concentrating, and say, 'Yes, I do remember you, but from where?' If that doesn't work, I tell them they look twenty years younger, and ask if they've had work done."

THE VANISHING NOTION

Another type of blocking—when an entire concept disappears before you can get it out of your mouth—is also very intimidating. "You can hear it in people's conversations," observes Karen, the grant writer. "I call it the 'fluttering butterfly.' Someone's in the middle of a sentence, and suddenly it's 'And so, yeah, uh, I, um.' You can see it in her eyes—she's forgotten everything." Because scientists have been unable to establish a guaranteed method of making subjects lose their trains of thought (they might want to consider replicating the conditions in my kitchen at 6:00 P.M. on a school night), no one has studied this disconcerting phenomenon in a laboratory. (There is a world of difference, by the way, between what scientists can study in a laboratory setting—for instance, the ability to memorize a string of unrelated words—and the kind of thing that goes on in real life, such as remembering a list of items to buy at the market. It's not clear that the former generalizes to the latter, but for now, it's the best researchers can do.) In the case of the disappearing concept, it seems evident that powerful interference is involved: Something has thrown you off target—the look on your boss's face, an eager waiter, a sketchy idea you intended to include—and then it's all gone. Bonnie, a political fund-raiser, reports that she "totally blanked in the middle of a speech" while lecturing before a large group. "I could not remember a single point that I wanted to make. No matter how hard I tried, my brain just fizzled. Finally I had to just be quiet and encourage someone else to take the floor." To retrieve an idea that has gone AWOL demands stealth. You sneak up on it, working backward from where you were when you lost it to some brand-new inspiration.

A distinct, and frightening type of blocking occurs when you find that you're totally lost in a neighborhood you know well. "A few years ago," wrote Sean, the information technology specialist, "I was driving in my hometown when I lost my bearings, as if I'd been plopped down in a strange area. What road was I on? How far from home? What if I turned right or left? I was clueless. It must have lasted twenty seconds or longer, which is not long by ordinary standards, but an eternity when you're lost like that, knowing that the streets ought to look familiar."

DO I KNOW YOU?

It is normal, though unpleasant, to encounter the occasional mental brick wall. Not so normal, however, is another type of blocking, called prosopagnosia, which involves forgetting not only the name of the person who stands before you, but his entire identity. Arthur, a writer, confessed to me that he doesn't remember faces. (Neither do I, so he was in excellent company.)

"When I say that to people, they always say, 'Well, I don't remember names either.' And I say, 'No, you don't understand: I don't remember faces of people I've met fifty times.'" Before a party one evening, where he knew he would run into an editor he'd worked with for years, he panicked. "I'd met her several times, but mostly, we'd had a phone relationship." He could not call to mind any details of her appearance. "I walked into the party and I looked around and I wondered if she was there. I thought, Is she short or tall? Does she have brown hair? Somebody came up to me partway through the party and I was talking to her and I thought, Is this my editor? I just had no idea."

An executive told me that the day before a gala dinner, she'd conducted an hour-long private meeting with a man she wanted as a client. The next evening, at the event, she walked right past him, a move that he reasonably interpreted as the ultimate brush-off. Kim, a real estate broker in Milwaukee, with hundreds of clients, some of whom she hadn't seen in years, explained that she'd learned to enthusiastically embrace the total strangers who threw their arms around her. Victor, the economist, recalled his embarrassment on the Sunday in the mountains when he and his daughter took a lunch break after a morning of skiing and shared a table with an unfamiliar woman who knew his name and claimed that she had been his executive assistant for several years.

Prosopagnosia is a hurdle for me. I recognize very few celebrities, actors or world leaders, which makes me feel like a dolt. I can properly tag close friends and family, but identifying much of the rest of the world is tough. A large social event or a business meeting sets me on edge: Who will I forget? Who will I offend? Seeing her in some other context, I've been known to offer an enormous greeting to the supermarket cashier, but to walk right past the mother of one of my son's best friends. There are times when I behave in an awkward, formal manner in an effort to avoid revealing my shortcomings. I envy the chimps. They have better facial recognition skills than humans, and are particularly talented at recognizing faces when they're upside down.

For years I blamed myself. But in the course of my research, I learned that the persistent failure to recognize faces does not stem, as I'd darkly suspected, from an outrageous level of self-absorption. Prosopagnosia has neurological underpinnings. The lack of facial recognition is thought to be the result of abnormalities, damage or impairment in the right fusiform gyrus, a fold in the brain that appears to coordinate the neural systems that control facial perception and memory. Images of faces—the proportions and distances of eyes, nose, mouth, the color of hair—reside in one part of the brain, while the defining aspects of the face—the expressions in eyes and on lips, for instance—reside in another.

Cognitively normal people combine the two sources of data, allowing for the identification of thousands of people on sight. Prosopagnosic people do not. Frequent failures suggest brain injury or other neurological damage. I tucked that information in the back of my mind, certain that I'd remember to bring it up when I visited the UCLA Memory Clinic the following week.

5

INTO THE DOUGHNUT HOLE

. . .

What a Brain Scan Can (and Cannot) Tell You About What's Going on Upstairs

There are more linear feet of hallway in UCLA's Neuropsychological Institute than in the Pentagon, or at least that's the rumor. I walked down windowless corridors, looking for the solitary elevator that went to the eighth floor. I was sure that this was the place for me to take the first step in ruling out the biggest, scariest thing. In Gary Small's expert hands, I intended to quash the nagging fear that my forgetfulness, rather than reflecting the normal process of aging, was an early symptom of incipient Alzheimer's disease.

Gary Small, the psychiatrist who directs both the UCLA Center on Aging and the UCLA Memory Clinic, is the author of *The Memory Bible*, the book that earned him the title of Memory Maven and made him the darling of morning television. But for Small, turning out a book every couple of years is just an avocation. His real work involves developing imaging technology that he hopes will eventually allow doctors to diagnose Alzheimer's disease years before symptoms arise.

When we spoke on the phone several weeks earlier, I gave him the lowdown on my cognitive state. I told him that I'd taken the memory tests in his book and filled out the charts. "I scored in the range where you say a person ought to consult a doctor," I said. "I figured you were the man for the job."

I needed to know, I told him, where I fell on the spectrum. He'd explained that his team tries to sort out who is experiencing the normal sorts of losses you see with age, and who might be demonstrating the earliest manifestations of Alzheimer's disease and related dementias. His lab was at the vanguard of positron emission tomography (PET), a brain-scanning technology that allows nuclear-imaging specialists to observe the amount of metabolic activity present in different regions of the brain. Alzheimer's disease, he explained, produces a distinct and abnormal pattern of activity in the parietal and medial temporal lobes. On a PET scan, this stands out like a sore thumb. "The metabolic activity of brain cells changes very little with age," he said, "unless there is some pathology in place and the cells are weakening or dying."

When PET scanning was combined with functional magnetic resonance imaging (fMRI), which allowed researchers to see the relationship between metabolism and blood flow in the brain, as well as neuropsychological testing and blood work, Small's team could predict with 95 percent accuracy whether a patient would develop the symptoms of Alzheimer's disease within three years. The greatest gift he could offer anyone, he observed, was a clean bill of health.

I asked him whether he thought I had reason to be worried. "Is it progressive?" he asked. "Is the impairment you perceive getting worse?"

I couldn't say for sure what had changed in the last six months. Like everybody else, I was considerably less mentally agile than I was when I was thirty, when I could readily juggle several mental tasks at once. Maybe it was age, but maybe it wasn't.

I ought to be prepared, Small said, to learn something I might wish I didn't know. If I satisfied the requirements for participation in one of his research studies, I'd get a PET scan and an fMRI, and as part of the bargain, these would be read by scientists who arguably had analyzed more brain scans than anyone else on the planet. On the open market, these were pricey items—at least $3,000 for the duo. It sounded like a good deal to me.

THE GAP BETWEEN DISEASE AND DIAGNOSIS

There are two forms of Alzheimer's disease—familial and sporadic. It is still not clear how they are related—or whether they are actually two distinct conditions that produce similar pathology, like juvenile and type 2 diabetes. The familial strain, referred to as "early onset," emerges from hereditary genetic mutations, appearing while an individual is still in his thirties or forties. It is swift, merciless, and, luckily, extremely rare, accounting for only 5 percent of U.S. cases.

The sporadic form of the disease is the one we've come to know too well. After sixty-five, it afflicts one out of ten. By eighty, it's one in four. After eighty-five, it's nearly half. When I read those statistics, I assumed that sporadic Alzheimer's was a disease of late onset, appearing in old age.

Then I discovered studies suggesting that Alzheimer's actually began in midlife, decades before memory loss interfered with the activities of daily living. In the course of my research, I became acquainted with several middle-aged people who had recognized early on, when they still appeared perfectly competent to the rest of the world, that something was seriously amiss. They knew, long before anyone else suspected it, that their minds were changing in drastic ways. At sixty, Stuart, a surgeon, began forgetting the names of bones, organs and procedures he used every day in his work. At fifty-four, Bruce, a common-pleas judge, realized to his horror that he'd started to leave full lines out of his sentencing. Joanna, a family-law attorney, fifty-six, found that she was losing track of clients' names and the details of their cases. The fifty-four-year-old general counsel of a large entertainment company, Ralph, struggled fruitlessly to remain abreast of the workload he'd managed for over two decades. In their initial evaluation, these patients aced the neuropsychological test called the Mini-Mental State Exam that physicians typically administer to help diagnose memory disorders. The MMSE, as it is known, consists of thirty items that assess language, orientation, calculation, attention, recall and visuospatial function. Several studies have shown that the MMSE is sensitive only to overt dementia, but that hasn't stopped primary-care physicians—and some neurologists—from mistakenly giving it to obviously sentient patients who complain of memory loss.

When these healthy middle-aged patients initially presented perfect scores on the MMSE, their doctors attributed their symptoms to mood disorders, prescribing antidepressants and relaxing vacations, inadvertently wasting months during which they might have benefited from participation in clinical trials of new Alzheimer's drugs and other interventions.

Over months and years, as I got to know these people, I looked for similarities in their histories. (The general counsel died, at fifty-nine, before I met him. His daughter told me his story.) None of them fit the classic Alzheimer's profile—no one was obese or diabetic. No one had heart disease. They were not heavy drinkers or smokers. In fact, all four were preternaturally fit and focused on staying that way— the judge and the surgeon ran regular marathons and continued to do so well into their disease. The family-law attorney was an avid solo sailor; the general counsel had been a distance road biker. I searched for a common thread, a clue to what might have brought them down. Initially, I knew only that they were high-achieving people who had spent many years in relentlessly stressful, intellectually demanding careers. I'd encountered a lot of people like that. Come to think of it, I was a person like that. It was folly, I realized, to pretend that those of us in midlife had a free pass.

THE ASSESSMENT BEGINS

At the UCLA Memory Clinic, Small's research associate, Andrea Kaplan, greeted me and settled me at a small round table in the reception area. In the company of another middle-aged woman, presumably a patient at the clinic, I began to complete a bulky set of medical forms. How would I rate my memory right now, compared to how it was functioning a year ago? How could I be expected to give an accurate assessment? I sighed loudly, and the woman sitting next to me looked up from her own forms and offered a commiserating smile.

I filled out the psychological profile, describing how I felt at the moment. Did I feel calm? Pleasant? Anxious? I chose the last, wondering how many people who visited this office—where it was possible to learn very bad news—actually could achieve a tranquil state of mind. Another sheet, titled "General Frequency of Forgetting," asked how often I forgot names, faces, appointments, where I put things, or the thread of a conversation. How often did I forget whether or not I'd told somebody something? Did I have trouble recalling what I'd read a few sentences before? Did I ever forget that I'd left something on the stove, or blank on the ingredients in a recipe in the middle of assembling it? After I noted that all of these were frequent occurrences, I peeked at the page open in front of my tablemate. Quickly, she covered it with her forearm. I wanted to tell her that I was friend, not foe, that I was there preparing for Intervention #1 in the name of all of us.

I looked up to find Gary Small, dapper in a navy sports coat and natty tie, an amicable, wiry man of fifty. After a friendly chat, he turned me over to his deputy, Cody Wright, a psychiatrist so youthful in appearance that I wondered whether he actually knew what it felt like to walk into the kitchen and forget what you'd come for. In the exam room, Wright settled us both into chairs and ran through the questions that comprise the MMSE, which has been part of the standard diagnostic repertoire since it was introduced in 1975.

He requested that I tell him today's date, as well as the day of the week. He wanted to know the season, the state we were in, the city, and the neighborhood. He asked for the name of the building, and the floor we were on. Then he named three objects—street, banana and hammer—which he instructed me to remember. He'd quiz me on them later. He had me spell "world" backward, a task that required my fingers—"d...l...o." Then he told me to count backward from one hundred by sevens, a task over which I stumbled badly.

How did I know, he asked, that I had memory problems? I unleashed the litany, starting with the kitchen. Several times, I'd left the gas stove flaming for most of the day. I burned out the whistle in the teakettle, and then the bottom of the kettle itself, while answering e-mail. Summoned upstairs by a child who had misplaced a critical textbook, I'd puzzled over the burning smell coming from the kitchen, only to remember too late that I had been in the middle of making pancakes.

I'd exited the house through the garage, and left the front door wide open. I'd forgotten to lock the car, making us the target of burglars who pressed the button of the automatic garage-door opener clipped to the windshield visor and cleared out the contents of the first room they encountered, which happened to be my husband's office. They took his laptop, his backup drives, and our wall safe. He's a patient man, but it wasn't particularly good for our marriage.

Flipping through the sheaf of medical forms, Wright stopped at the section dedicated to sleep. I'd checked the box marked "poor" all the way down that column, but still, it was an understatement. I'd learned to wake up at the slightest noise when my kids were infants, I explained to him, and well over a decade later, my eyes still popped open at the sound of a pigeon on the roof or a snort from my sleeping husband. Four or five nights a week, I woke up at 3:00 A.M. Once my eyes were open, my mind was off to the races. If I fell asleep again, I snoozed for only a few minutes before the alarm clock went off. After a bad night, I felt abraded, as if my mind and body had been dragged across a sisal carpet.

"It's essential that you get the sleep thing handled," he said, scribbling some notes. He might as well have told me it was critical that I sprout wings. I'd tried all manner of natural remedies and pharmaceuticals. Melatonin worked for a week. Ambien worked for about three days before cutting out. Trazodone—an antidepressant that turned out, in clinical trials, to have such soporific side effects it was recast as a sleeping pill—worked very well indeed, but it left me sedated and bleary until lunchtime. Besides, I hated pills. For years, I'd prided myself on living without them. I didn't even take a multivitamin.

"How is your sense of direction?" Wright asked, rubbing his beardless chin. My internal compass had broken, I said. I'd traveled all over the world by myself, but now I had trouble reading a map while I was driving. I got lost going places I'd been several times before. I'd peer inside my head, waiting for the expected mental map to materialize, but the screen remained empty. When people gave me directions, on the street or in the gas station, I forgot what they told me almost before it was out of their mouths. Because I couldn't reverse directions in my mind, once I arrived at a place, I had trouble leaving it. "I used to make fun of people like me," I told him. "I thought they were wimps."

He checked his watch. We were due at the lab in a few minutes, and we still had six pages to cover. "Any manic episodes? Any changes in behavior or appearance? Any medications?" All negative. He wanted to know about my proclivity to panic (sometimes, when late and lost), my energy level (far too low for my life), irritability (just ask my husband), crying spells (oh, who has time?) and temper (the occasional flare-up). Did I own a weapon? Have suicidal thoughts? Had I ever had a head injury? "No," I told him, "none of those."

We rushed through the windowless halls to the lab, where Eunah, a friendly young nurse, handed me a gown and suggested that I stretch out on a hospital bed. She hooked me up for an EKG, then inserted a catheter into my bold green vein and extracted vial after vial of blood from my arm. I'd get the full workup. They'd check my calcium, iron, glucose and electrolyte levels, as well as kidney, liver and endocrine function. If any of these turned up out of normal range, it would help explain what was wrong with my memory.

INTO THE SCANNER

Ten days later, I learned that my tests were fine, at least so far. I could move forward, into stage two. Andrea Kaplan, Small's research associate, scheduled me for a PET scan, an fMRI and a stretch of neuropsych testing. Normally, these evaluations were conducted over two or three sequential visits. I'd complete them in six hours so that I could catch the evening plane back to Oakland. Kaplan warned me not to be late: Five research studies shared the PET scanner, and securing time on it required negotiation skills worthy of the United Nations.

As soon as I walked through the door, a graduate student escorted me to the PET scanner in the basement. Repeatedly, the attendant behind the counter in the waiting area answered the phone "pet department," making me think of dog bones and squeaky toys. Briefly, that diverted me from dwelling on what was to come.

I wasn't worried about the scan itself—not the ninety minutes of immobilization, or the needles in my arms, or the radioactive isotopes that were about to enter my body. What disquieted me was the realization that I'd set something in motion that I was now powerless to stop. If regions of my scan, instead of coming up in healthy, vivid colors, displayed more muted tones that signified abnormal glucose metabolism, my future prospects would be irrevocably changed.

Three years before, Joanna, the family-law attorney, stood on this same speckled linoleum floor, under the same fluorescent lights, and contemplated a giant cream-colored PET scanner with "Siemens ECAT" emblazoned on the surface. At fifty-six, she was on the verge of becoming a judge. The little law firm she'd started twenty years earlier had grown successful enough to support two partners. It provided her with a beautiful house in Orange County and a boat that she loved to sail solo over choppy open water to Santa Catalina Island. She had enough money to help out her two adult kids, and she was in love with Theo, a slender, handsome, sparkly-eyed man two decades her senior, whom she'd met on a private sailboat cruise off the waters of Turkey.

It would have been perfect if she hadn't suspected she was losing her mind. In early 2000, she began to have difficulty remembering her clients. She struggled over basic aspects of the law. Her physicians—an internist and two neurologists—told her that her problem was related to menopause, depression or stress. She was far too young, and much too high functioning, to have developed Alzheimer's disease. They offered up the old saw, apparently a staple in medical school classrooms of the 1970s: "The person with Alzheimer's disease is not the one who forgot where he parked the car; he's the one who forgot that he came in a car." They reassured her that people with Alzheimer's had no idea they were forgetting things. That Joanna was concerned about her memory was therefore evidence that everything was just fine.

The neurologists supported their conclusions with her perfect scores on the MMSE, which, as I mentioned before, is sensitive to overt dementia, but entirely blind to early symptoms. She prayed that the doctors were right, and that her difficulties would abate, but her condition grew worse. In 2001, after reading about UCLA's diagnostic success, she arranged to go there for a full evaluation.

Normally, the results would have been sent to a referring physician, who would have broken the news. Because she'd arrived at UCLA without a referral, Joanna's results went straight to her, over her office fax. "Diagnosis consistent with Alzheimer's disease" was at the top of the page. Her partner and her employees knew at the same time she did. Joanna, always physically robust, assumed she'd practice law until she was in her seventies. Once she was diagnosed, her partner, who had been her best friend for over thirty years, told her that whether or not she felt capable of continuing to practice, no one would hire an attorney with Alzheimer's disease. She had to resign from the firm. She had no retirement plan, no disability insurance and no long-term-care policy.

I was thinking about Joanna when the imaging technician announced that he had patients stacked up in the hallways like it was Christmas Eve at LAX. It was time to get started. He eased me into the scanner bed, encouraging me to slide my head up toward the doughnut hole. He slipped a foam bolster beneath my knees, but the bed itself was a rock-hard half-pipe, barely wide enough to contain me. He carefully positioned my head. Then, with a flourish, he pulled some hardware-store masking tape off a fat roll and wrapped it around my cranium, securing my head to the cradle. "This is our high-tech method," he joked. "We tried everything else, but nothing works so well." He set the laser line, positioning my brain in the crosshairs. When he pushed a button, sending the half-pipe into the doughnut hole, I entered a beige, featureless world. "Perfect," he said. "Don't move or the next hour will be wasted."

The machine made a purring, gurgling noise that was actually soothing. I'd have slept except that I knew what came next—the part with the needles. A nurse prepped one arm to receive FDG, the radioactive isotope that would enter my bloodstream and rapidly cross the blood-brain barrier. The PET scan measured the rate that glucose was taken up by brain cells, which would indicate how effectively the cells were functioning and communicating. The other arm, the one I'd shortly wish I could use to scratch my nose, was catheterized so that I could provide three test tubes of blood, one every fifteen minutes. The samples would be spun in the on-site lab, to make sure that the isotope, which had a short half-life, was leaving my bloodstream on schedule.

When the technician returned to release me from bondage, he ripped the masking tape off my head and hustled me off the table. He apologized, explaining that they needed this scanner right that second. The other one had malfunctioned, after they'd already injected a patient with the radioactive isotope. I grabbed my shoes and greeted my graduate student, who guided me to the cafeteria. She waited patiently while I bought myself a turkey sandwich on whole wheat with extra pickles, and rushed me back up to the eighth floor for my neuropsychological testing.

WORD PAIRS AND PUZZLES

A full battery of neuropsychological tests takes two days and can cost several thousand dollars. The tests measure general intellect, executive function, sequencing, reasoning, problem solving, attention and con-centration, learning and memory, language, visual-spatial skills, motor and sensory skills, as well as mood and personality. At UCLA, I was going to have the quickie assessment, just to make sure that I wasn't seriously out of whack—forty-five minutes, tops.

"You'd better eat some of that sandwich before we get started," said Claudia, the doctoral candidate who sat behind the desk, flip charts poised. As soon as I'd made a dent in my lunch, she read me a brief story, a neuropsych classic, about a robbery victim, a woman who worked as a cook in a restaurant. It was packed with details, and soon after she finished reading, she asked me to repeat as many of them as I could. I believed I'd paid close attention, but in truth, I recalled very little. This scared me to death. My career as a journalist was built on my ability to accurately recall facts. What did it mean if I could not remember the street on which the woman lived, or even her name?

We moved on to other tasks. A few were easy: I nailed a list of vocabulary word definitions. I could readily name common objects when I was shown pictures. My recall of a list of verbal pairs was deemed "superior." But it took me five tries to recall and repeat all fifteen words the evaluator read to me from a list. She showed me an abstract figure that looked something like a rocket ship and asked me to copy it, which was easy enough. When she removed the figure, and asked me to draw it from memory, the only thing I drew was a blank. Equally daunting was a stint at the computer screen, where I was supposed to grasp an overriding "rule" that apparently existed in the groupings of various geometric figures. I couldn't find it. I felt oddly dizzy and lost. I knew I was making a hash of things.

When I saw Andrea Kaplan standing in the doorway, I breathed a sigh of relief. I was ready to collapse, I told her. That was fine, she said. The MRI I was about to have required only that I lie still.

"You mean the fMRI, right?" I was looking forward to seeing my brain in action.

She shook her head sadly. The brand-new, state-of-the art fMRI machine, installed in its own custom-built lodgings, was still not op-erative. Physicists were working on it, day and night, but so far, no luck. This was extremely disappointing, and had required the last-minute revision of several research protocols. For now, the MRI machine would have to do. So instead of gaining insight into my brain's function, I would see only its structure.

Compared to the PET scanner, the MRI machine was a suite in a luxury hotel. The bed was cushioned and sheeted, the room was cool, the lights were low. The technician asked if I had a pacemaker or any other internal metal fittings, which would have been catastrophically attracted to the powerful magnet. He told me to remove all my jewelry. Gently, he helped me climb onboard, offered me earplugs and sent me backward into the opening. Inside, there was a strategically placed mirror that allowed me to see the technician in the booth, flipping his switches. Then, the noise began—BAM BAM BAM BAM BAM, like the first driving notes of a heavy-metal song. I waited expectantly for the break, but it never came. Eventually, I had to abandon the music metaphor and accept the fact that I had a hardworking carpenter in there with me, driving nails. Somehow, I fell asleep.

Forty-five minutes later, the technician woke me. Would I like to see what my brain looked like on the computer monitor? He showed me a moonlike landscape, replete with crevasses and ridges, dark seas and deep valleys. Curious and possessive, I was as drawn to it as I was to my unborn child's first sonogram. "There are the frontal lobes," he said, "and there are the hippocampi," pointing to a pair of gentle crescents deep in the middle of the brain. I pulled closer to the monitor. In front of me on the screen was everything that makes me who I am.

Ten days later, Gary Small told me that the news was great. I'd passed every test. My PET scan was as good as gold—the pattern of distribution for the FDG isotope was symmetrical and unremarkable. My MRI showed no sign of atrophy in the grooves called sulci, or the bumps called gyri. The ventricles—the spaces in the brain that are filled with cerebrospinal fluid—were the perfect size. I was clear of any indications of Alzheimer's disease, a prognosis that currently came with only a three-year guarantee, but was likely, Small said, to be good for much longer. I was a fine candidate, he noted, for one of his current studies, the 14-Day Memory Prescription Program. He was getting terrific results. One guy's verbal memory had doubled. He hoped I'd participate.

"What about the neuropsych evaluation?" I asked, remembering my sense of abject failure. He spoke carefully: I'd had a range of tests. When the results were averaged, I fell within the normal range for my age and education. At the time, I thought that sounded fine.

"That's a great relief," I said to Small.

"A lot of people feel that way," he said modestly.

It was helpful to have the three-year, "free and clear" promise, and I left UCLA with a bounce in my step. Slowly, over the next few months, I began to realize that there was a lot more to learn. Although PET and MRI neuroimaging were useful tools for sniffing out Alzheimer's pathology already so well established that the patient displayed frank symptoms, the earliest signs of the disease—the slow aggregation of proteins—remained invisible to scanning technology. What Gary Small did not address were the myriad other explanations for the development of midlife cognitive deficits.

It was time to move on.

6

SWALLOW THIS

• • •

The Feeding of a Midlife Brain:

Essential Fatty Acids, Vitamins,

Supplements and Plenty of Glucose

I'd scratched my head over study after study, trying to decide if there was any merit in swallowing a Ziploc bag full of vitamins each morning. Surely, some of those tablets and capsules would do me good, but which ones? In my part of northern California, vitamin stores and holistic pharmacies fill shelf after shelf with products that promise, however vaguely, to "support" memory and attention. The claims are unsubstantiated and the products unregulated. "I take millions of vitamins and drink green tea and nothing helps," said Ryan, a movie producer. Even if your heart is fine, recent studies suggest that you may have wasted your money. In supplement form, most antioxidants—including vitamin E, vitamin C and beta carotene—show no protective effect. It's safe to say that antioxidants only mop up free radicals (their main job) when you consume them in the real McCoy—fruits and vegetables. Why this is remains unclear, but researchers suspect that in supplement form, antioxidants are digested and absorbed too quickly. When you eat fruits and vegetables, the fiber keeps them in the digestive system for a longer stretch, maximizing their benefits.

Despite these vagaries, Americans lay out over $23 billion a year on dietary supplements. Of that figure, about $210 million is spent on micronutrients promoted as aids to mental acuity. On ginkgo biloba, for which little evidence of effectiveness exists, sales exceed $1 billion. Those who spend money on brain boosters are not typically elderly, observes Don Summerfield, cofounder of Pharmaca, a group of nine integrative pharmacies in the western United States. They're middle-aged people who feel enormous pressure to keep up the pace.

This interest in improving memory through supplementation isn't new. The ancient Greeks, whose oral tradition demanded that they keep track of some very long poems, were inclined to wreathe their heads in rosemary and sniff lemon balm on days that were expected to be cognitively demanding. Aristotle preferred to apply a compound of weasel, beaver and mole fat, presumably to his scalp, although records are vague. For 3,500 years, the Chinese have addressed memory issues with boiled decoctions that combine the benefits of many herbs. Indian practitioners of ayurvedic medicine have treated cognitive impairment since the sixth century with syrups intended to enhance concentration, creativity and working memory. In India, the use of *Bacopa monieri*—a dried plant nicknamed Brahmi because it opens the gate of Brahma, or intelligence—is centuries old and remains widespread. Parents and grandparents take it to maintain their own brain function, but they also give it to schoolchildren to improve their performance on fiercely competitive exams.

A BRAIN-FRIENDLY DIET

Except during my pregnancies, when I managed to choke down a horse-size vitamin pill every day for the sake of my unborn child, I'd carefully avoided vitamins. Then I read about Carl Cotman's study of elderly beagles. Cotman, the director of the University of California, Irvine's Institute of Brain Aging and Dementia, had been working with these hounds for years. They were interesting, he said, because they suffered a decline in memory that closely resembled the symptomatology of Alzheimer's disease. Cotman compared a group of dogs who maintained an active lifestyle (social interaction, new toys every day) and ate a diet of standard dog chow, enriched with foods high in vitamins and antioxidants (tomatoes, carrot granules, citrus pulp and spinach flakes) to dogs who had equivalent social benefits and toys, but a regular diet. The enriched diet was fortified with vitamin E and vitamin C, as well as two other supplements, alpha-lipoic acid and acetyl-L-carnitine. As the study progressed, researchers tested the dogs with a series of increasingly difficult learning problems. Three-quarters of the dogs in the supplemented diet/active lifestyle group were able to perform the tasks successfully. The dogs in the control group, the ones who ate a standard diet, were mostly mystified. "We can basically improve learning and memory in these aged animals, so that they can do more complicated tasks and make fewer mistakes," noted Cotman. He'd not only slowed the aging process in these dogs, he'd started to reverse it.

If this worked so conclusively for an elderly beagle, maybe it was worth my time. At Gary Small's invitation, I enrolled in the human version of Cotman's beagle trial, the 14-Day Memory Prescription Program, designed to ascertain whether improved nutrition and increased exercise, in addition to stress reduction and memory training, would quickly result in cognitive improvements.

Back in Los Angeles, I met with Deborah Dorsey, the UCLA Center on Aging's registered nurse. Quite formally, she placed a thick blue binder on the table before me. For two weeks, she said, I would live by its dictates. I shouldn't kid myself, she said: With two sons to care for and a book to write, this was going to be hard work.

Briefly, we discussed my diet. Although more than half our grocery budget went to fresh fruits and vegetables, I knew that my consumption fell far short of the five to nine servings of fruits and vegetables that the USDA recommended. I couldn't figure out how anyone managed to get that many down, I told her.

The program would get me on the right track, she said. I'd receive the proper balance of protein and carbohydrates, as well as sufficient quantities of antioxidants and essential fatty acids. Each day, I'd take a multivitamin with 400 micrograms of folate, as well as an additional 400 IUs of vitamin E, 1,000 milligrams of vitamin C (500 in the morning, 500 in the evening) and 1,000 milligrams of an omega-3 fatty acid supplement in the form of fish oil. I'd have to stick close to the paring knife, the cutting board and the stove, in order to provide the three requisite meals and three snacks per day. She paged through the blue binder, stopping at the grocery list, which was four pages long. A quick scan of the first week's plan told me I'd be getting up earlier than usual—how else could I prepare the chopped-vegetable omelet with one yolk and two whites? I'd be eating quite a bit more protein at breakfast and lunch than was my custom. Protein yields glucose more slowly and reliably than fruits and vegetables, so it's valuable as a source of long-term fuel. Even the snacks involved prep time. Before I could leave the house, I'd stuff a Ziploc bag full of raw cut veggies, and somehow pack a cup of bouillon to go. Nutrition was only one aspect of the 14-Day Memory Prescription Program. I'd do different physical exercises each day and put my brain to work memorizing pairs of words and faces. There were brainteasers and mind-benders. Frankly, I was a little afraid of them.

I'd been on Gary Small's program for less than a week when it hit me. For most of my adult life, I'd been starving my neurons. Since my early twenties, I'd had only a cup of tea in the morning, until I was sure I had squeezed every viable word from my brain. I waited for lunch until I was so light-headed I could barely find the refrigerator, and then nibbled absentmindedly at my desk while I continued to work. Dinner, which I perceived as my just reward for the denial that had preceded it, was very large. Usually, I returned for seconds.

Stupidly, I'd been depriving my brain of glucose, its basic fuel. Even my lunch, usually a salad, yielded very little brain food—leafy greens, as healthy as they are, consist primarily of dietary fiber, which passes through the body undigested. That bleary feeling that you get when you're hungry has a cellular basis: Without enough glucose, the mitochondria, which function as the cell's power source, have nothing to burn, and the body's metabolic rate dips by 15 or 20 percent.

In youth, a couple of bites of a peanut butter sandwich can restore glucose levels, but older brains, which suffer more than younger ones from a glucose shortage, take more time to return to full function. Because blood levels of glucose influence how reliably neurons release acetylcholine, the neurotransmitter most involved in learning and memory, it's likely that you'll have more trouble recalling factual information that you try to absorb when your stomach is empty.

The memory prescription regimen of three meals and three snacks a day instantly made me feel smarter. In addition to increasing my intake of lean protein, the program's diet emphasized complex carbohydrates, among them oatmeal, brown rice, whole grain pasta, barley, bulgur, wheat berries and millet. These break down slowly, allowing glucose to be released into the bloodstream over an extended period. Carbohydrates consist entirely of chains of sugar molecules. Simple sugars—the ones that break down fast and leave you feeling dull—are made up of just one or two sugar molecules. Complex carbs may contain hundreds of simple sugar molecules, joined together. Once complex carbs are in your stomach, digestive enzymes break them down into single glucose molecules that can pass through the intestinal wall. Leftover glucose, for which the body has no immediate need, is stored as glycogen and released under conditions of physiological stress.

AVOIDING BRAIN RUST

On Gary Small's program, I ate so many fruits and vegetables that I may have actually met the USDA recommendations. These, Dorsey assured me, were high in antioxidants. I'd heard the term, of course, but like most people, I had no idea why consuming tons of them would be important for my brain.

I phoned James Joseph, the director of the neuroscience lab at the Human Nutrition Center at Tufts University. His study of rats that were fed extract of blueberries for eight weeks had made headlines all over the world. They showed marked declines in oxidative stress, as well as improved memory and concentration. (In rats, such abilities are measured by how efficiently they get through a maze to find a food reward.)

I asked Joseph to explain why this had worked. Free radicals, he observed, which are oxygen molecules, arise as part of the essential metabolic process. Such molecules seek to bond with electrons, which they scavenge from other cells. Any nearby molecule—fat, protein, even DNA—will do. This process goes on throughout life, Joseph explained, but in youth, our genes are fairly good at repairing the damage. By the time we reach middle age, those repair genes are less efficient, and we begin to develop a sort of internal rusting, called oxidative stress.

I told Joseph that I'd just purchased three boxes of blueberries at a staggering pre-season high of $5.99 each, in order to conform to the requirements of my new memory prescription diet. "Well, don't tell anybody," he said, "but I get the flash-frozen ones, unless I'm up in Maine in August. In the winter, what's coming in is from Chile, and I can't say how those are shipped or handled or packaged. If they're not stored where it's cold enough, you can kiss those antioxidants good-bye."

For years, nutritionists have advocated the "rainbow on the plate" approach, proposing that deeply hued fruits and vegetables pack the most oxidative punch. More recent research suggests that several fruits and vegetables that adorn themselves in quiet neutrals, including onions, artichokes and russet potatoes, are also excellent sources of antioxidants. Spices such as cinnamon and curcumin (the yellow pigment found in turmeric, a key seasoning in curry) make the top five of the *Journal of Agriculture and Food Chemistry*'s antioxidant list. Research shows that Indians who eat large amounts of curry develop Alzheimer's disease at barely a quarter the rate of Americans, suggesting that the spice—and a fish- and vegetable-heavy, meat-free diet—actually does some good. Peanuts (straight from the shells, with pinkish skins intact), pecans and almonds are also powerful antioxidants. Red wine, grape juice and pomegranate juice are hailed for their protective properties, as are green and black tea and dark chocolate. Recently, apples and apple juice got a five-star endorsement for their antioxidant qualities. The proverb, "An apple a day keeps the doctor away," may have something to it: Mice on an apple-rich diet performed significantly better on a maze test and showed elevated levels of the neurotransmitter acetylcholine, critical to learning and memory. Human trials will begin soon, but researchers think that two 8-ounce glasses of apple juice or two to three apples a day may do the trick.

WHY YOU NEED ESSENTIAL FATTY ACIDS

The 14-Day Memory Prescription Program's diet also boosted my consumption of essential fatty acids (EFAs), especially omega-3s. In the body, omega-3s subdivide into two fatty acids, DHA and EPA. DHA is particularly important because it provides the perfect raw material for building healthy brain cell membranes. About 40 percent of midlife Americans are deficient in essential fatty acids, which are critical for optimal neuronal function. EFAs comprise the raw material of myelin, the covering of lipid fat that surrounds a neuron's delicate branches. They also form the cell membrane, which maintains a neuron's structural integrity. EFAs make the membrane more fluid and flexible, allowing the cell to be more receptive to incoming signals. In addition, recent research suggests that they facilitate the production of brain-derived neurotropic factor, which engenders the growth of new cells.

Like most of us, I assumed that I could satisfy my essential fatty acids requirement by eating a nice four-ounce fillet of wild salmon about once a week. In reality, to maintain an adequate supply, I'd need two or three times that much fatty, cold-water fish. As I'll discuss in Chapter 14, there are reasons not to eat that much fish in a single week.

Other sources of essential fatty acids are almonds, pecans, soybeans, walnuts, flaxseeds and avocados, although the body doesn't absorb them as readily as the EFAs in seafood. Fish oil supplements, once hailed as a good way to increase EFAs, are now suspected of containing dangerous levels of methyl mercury. Because EFAs are so desirable, there's a movement afoot to pump them into foods that don't naturally contain them as additives to eggs, soy milk and bread. According to a recent report from the University of Pittsburgh, scientists are working on engineering transgenic pigs, intended to yield meat that's full of EFAs. You'd have to eat five enriched eggs, each containing around 190 milligrams of EFAs, to match the benefit available in a three-ounce serving of salmon. The bread's no bargain, either: To get comparable quantities, you'd need to eat twenty-four slices.

Traditionally, the EFAs we consumed in staples like fish or nuts accounted for most of our intake of dietary fat. In the latter half of the twentieth century, as processed foods began to dominate the culinary landscape, trans fat crept into the diet, and into the molecules that make up our cells. Trans fats grew popular because they make foods resistant to rancidity and allow grocers to keep them on the shelves for an extended period. Because trans-fat oils can be heated and cooled repeatedly, they are fast-food restaurants' number one choice for frying. Essential fatty acids allow the cell membrane to remain flexible because of a natural curve in their molecular structure. In contrast, trans-fat molecules are straighter, narrower and more rigid. When your diet contains more trans fats than EFAs, the trans-fat molecules slip into EFA slots. Because the stiffer trans-fat molecules in neurons don't conduct chemically driven nerve impulses nearly as well as EFAs, the speed at which you process information is gradually reduced. Trans fats can get in the way of the metabolism of essential fatty acids, and can also lead to insulin resistance, which, as I'll discuss in Chapter 16, presents a significant problem for a large percentage of the middle-aged population.

The good news is that if you increase your consumption of EFAs and greatly reduce or eliminate trans fats, your neuronal cell membranes will recover. Regretting every trans-fat-laden commercially baked chocolate chip cookie and piece of squishy sandwich bread I ever ate, I was anxious to hurry the process along.

For a full two weeks, while I participated in Gary Small's program, I ate admirably. I endured the looks I received from my children and husband when I set down yet another bowl of brown rice or served the vegetables without the customary pat of butter. We all knew it would come to an end, if only because I don't have the necessary hours available in my life to accomplish the constant shopping and chopping, packing and toting. No one in my family is a hard-core fast-food fan, but on a busy night after a crazy day, I need to be able to push a frozen lasagna into the oven and call it dinner.

I suspected that there might be an easier way. I knew that it was better to get the bulk of your nutrients from good, fresh food—but wasn't there some product that bundled up all the micronutrients and made it simple? After considerable research, I came upon an all-in-one product called Brain Sustain, developed by a board-certified neurologist, David Perlmutter, who is the author of *The Better Brain Book*. Every ingredient is listed on the label, and on iNutritional's Web site, where a month's supply costs $58.50. It was simple enough: You made yourself a smoothie, added two scoops of Brain Sustain and slugged it down. It cost a couple of dollars a day, and with the exception of magnesium, which is not water soluble, it contained everything I needed. (The magnesium is important: Researchers at MIT recently found that 420 milligrams for males and 320 milligrams for females helps maintain the plasticity of nerve cells, as well as several levels of neurotransmitters. Up to 80 percent of people in the United States are magnesium deficient, a condition which may result in a short attention span, confusion, memory loss, insomnia, mood changes, apathy and fatigue.)

I still wasn't sure that a one-size-fits-all solution, however handy, would fit me. Melanie Haiken, who often writes about nutrition for health magazines, let me take a peek at her medicine cabinet. She takes twelve to fifteen vitamins and supplements each day, for her thyroid condition as well as for her high blood pressure, PMS, anxiety and cognitive issues. "I try to focus on a couple of issues at a time," she said. "Some of the supplements recommended for anxiety have sedative properties, which means that instead of sharpening you up, they put you to sleep." It was important to get the blend just right, she said. If she could manage that cocktail, I figured I could go a step further and get myself something custom-made.

IN THE HANDS OF THE GURU

In preparation for Intervention #2, I made an appointment with complementary medicine guru Dharma Singh Khalsa. Early in my research, I'd come upon his book, *Brain Longevity*, a comprehensive guide to vitamins, other supplements and drugs intended to improve mental acuity. Since then, he'd become quite well known for his aggressive approach to treating fading memory and attention. With his vanity-label vitamins and his many books and tapes, Khalsa had become a cottage industry. When the well-known preventive medicine specialist Andrew Weil answered questions about memory on his Web site, he referenced Khalsa as the source of his information.

The first time I met Khalsa, we had lunch in a café near his office in Tucson. In brilliant April sunshine, his face flushed pink under his turban, he told me his story. He was an American Sikh, born in Ohio and raised in Florida. He'd adopted his faith, his name, his white clothing and his turban after a spiritual awakening at the hands of a master yogi in New Mexico, who also introduced him to his wife, Kirti. When we parted, after a brief conversation in which I described my memory troubles and he discussed the success that he'd had in treating patients who came to him from all over the world, he grasped me firmly by the shoulders. I should not wait much longer, he cautioned me. Improvement was possible, he said, but I needed to understand that every day I wasted was one I would not regain.

I allowed half a year to slip by before I called him again. I knew I wanted aggressive treatment, but I was a little bit afraid. How much was too much? Some new data suggested that taking antioxidants in supplement form (rather than getting them from food sources) might upset the balance of free radicals and antioxidants, discouraging the body from calling up its own foot soldiers in the war against oxidation. Still, I wanted to hear it from an expert, a physician who had been fine-tuning brains for years. It took a while to set a date for a consultation. Khalsa was lecturing, he was writing, he was traveling in Europe.

When we met again, on a cold, gray day in February, Khalsa beamed at me over a scraggly white beard. Around his neck, he wore a large amethyst medallion on a thick gold chain. We spent several hours together, talking about diet, exercise and meditation. He felt that long, solitary walks and daily meditation were key to my recovery. I was doubtful. I already walked almost daily (fast, with dogs). And meditation, when I'd tried it, had been a bust—I always fell asleep. After I agreed to put in my best effort, he began to describe the vitamin and supplement plan he had in mind. He'd write prescriptions for several pharmaceutical-grade supplements, which I'd get from a compounding pharmacy. He'd order 10-milligram capsules of extended-release DHEA, a hormone synthesized from yams and soybeans. In humans, the adrenal glands produce DHEA, but as you age, levels of the hormone decline. My level was on the low side for my age, which Khalsa thought could account for my troubles. "I'm going to send you back up to the level of a twenty-five-year-old," he said. He'd seen strong cognitive benefits in women who were approaching the age of menopause.

Next on the list was coenzyme Q-10, one of the few antioxidants that is fat soluble, which means that it can rapidly cross the cell membrane, the better to protect against free radicals. It worked best, he said, when taken in combination with another antioxidant, alpha-lipoic acid. I'd take a golden capsule from the compounding pharmacy that contained 100 milligrams of each. I knew about alpha-lipoic acid, I told Khalsa excitedly—that was one of the supplements that Carl Cotman gave his elderly beagles.

Each day, I'd take six of his Longevity Gold Cap multivitamins, he said, three at breakfast and three at lunch. I thought I could hold off on that one, I said—I was still working on a king-size bottle of Centrum Silver I'd purchased for the 14-Day Memory Prescription

Program. "That's worthless," he scoffed. "Supermarket vitamins are intended to satisfy recommended dietary allowances. They're meant to avoid specific vitamin deficiencies so, for instance, you don't develop rickets. They do not reflect the dosage levels required for optimum health. If you want to make improvements to the state of the brain, you need more."

What made for a multivitamin that was worth taking? Foremost, he said, a good multivitamin must have substantial amounts of the full range of B vitamins. They are required for the conversion of glucose to energy. B-12 is essential for the formation and maintenance of myelin, the fatty covering on axons. A deficit in B-1, the vitamin called thiamine, results in a decline in the production of the memory-boosting neurotransmitter acetylcholine. Niacin, also a B vitamin, appears to be important in stemming mental decline. Folic acid (also known as folate) protects against a decline in spatial skills and verbal fluency, according to a Tufts University study. In a large Dutch investigation, elderly subjects took twice the RDA for folate, 800 micrograms per day. On average, their scores on cognitive tests were comparable to people 5.5 years younger. When folic acid combines with B-12, it breaks down the amino acid known as homocysteine. Elevated homocysteine levels have a deadly effect on the endothelial cells that line the arteries, promoting atherosclerosis, the hardening of the arteries of the heart and the brain, and consequently diminishing cerebral blood flow. High blood levels of homocysteine correlate with decreased performance levels on most cognitive tests.

For many years, scientists maintained that vitamin E protected against cancer, heart disease and dementia. In a 2004 study, Peter Zandi, a researcher at the Johns Hopkins School of Public Health, produced results from an observational study that suggested, in the strongest possible way, that a combination of 1,000 IUs of vitamin C and 1,000 IUs of vitamin E, taken together, protected against the pathological changes of Alzheimer's disease. That was thrilling news, especially for Khalsa, who had for years believed in the efficacy of the duo. In March 2005, however, the *Journal of the American Medical Association* announced study results showing that large doses of vitamin E actually increased the risk of congestive heart failure, and that in terms of preventing dementia, it was no better than a placebo. It was a disappointing result, Khalsa acknowledged, but it was important to remember that the individuals who participated in this study did not start with a clean slate—they were already suffering from various pathologies. Khalsa's vote remained firmly with vitamins E and C, at four times the RDA.

In addition, I'd take Longevity Brain Caps, packed with ginkgo biloba. Although evidence for gingko's effectiveness is marginal, it has a great many fans; in Germany, it's a $400 million prescription drug business, and it's nearly always the first drug prescribed for patients who may be developing Alzheimer's disease. Current thinking on gingko, presented in the *Journal of the American Medical Association* in 2002, suggests that it doesn't produce measurable benefits in healthy adults, but is only effective when the problem is poor blood circulation. Khalsa's Brain Caps also contained fish oil (mercury-free, he assured me) and phosphatidyl serine, known as PS, which theoretically bolsters the strength and flexibility of the cell membrane. It may also increase the production of a gene-activating chemical that helps facilitate the long-term consolidation of memory.

Khalsa explained that this was only a starting point. There were other paths we could travel. The amino acid called acetyl-L-carnitine, which transports energy-producing nutrients across the mitochondrial membrane, worked very well for some people. There was also vinpocetine, made from the periwinkle plant, which, like gingko biloba, increased blood circulation in the capillaries of the brain. He guessed that I'd find acetyl-L-carnitine or vinpocetine too stimulating. "I consider each person experimental," he said. "You never know exactly what will happen. I have a friend who took vinpocetine, and the next morning, he found that he'd driven all the way from Tucson to Apache Canyon, New Mexico," a distance of about five hundred miles.

My monthly tab for vitamins and supplements, including the items that were shipped to me from the compounding pharmacy, topped $125. That seemed like a fortune, until I considered what I routinely pay for a massage or a haircut, neither of which are expected to have long-term benefits. Dutifully, I sorted vitamins into Ziploc bags, which was actually a lot of work, and carried them with me everywhere I went. Within a couple of weeks, I noticed that I'd been sleeping better. It might have been the placebo effect, but I was out cold by ten o'clock and rarely awake before six in the morning. Like a contented hen, my disposition smoothed out. It wasn't as easy to ruffle my feathers. After a couple of months, whatever was keeping me in dreamland stopped working, and the raw, unbuffered feeling that accompanies sleep deprivation returned. For a while, I was so disappointed that I tossed the Ziploc bags and the nearly full plastic bottles in the back of the refrigerator and tried to forget about them. Finally, I decided that there was no point in letting them go to waste, and began gulping and swallowing once again. It couldn't hurt, I told myself. But I knew I was not out of the woods.

7

MENTAL AEROBICS

· · ·

From Tedious to Addictive:

Options for Exercising Your Neurons

As politely as possible, I suggested to Gary Small that his mental aerobics, although arguably effective for older, retired persons, were destined to piss off individuals in the throes of midlife. Each day of the fourteen-day program, I dedicated five to ten minutes each morning and evening to some mental challenge, like remembering a list of word pairs or solving a visual puzzle. No matter how intently I tried to concentrate on the matter at hand, my attention was elsewhere. No task in that blue binder was compelling enough to hold my interest, not when there was work to be done and the question of how to be in two places at once later that afternoon remained unresolved. Try as I might to focus on solving puzzles replete with boxes and arrows, number sequences and letter rearrangements, like many midlife adults, I'd lost the ability to turn out the lights on the distractions around me.

In a follow-up discussion at UCLA, I told Deborah Dorsey, the Center on Aging's registered nurse, that I'd had such little success with mental aerobics that I feared I would skew the study's results. She wasn't reassuring. Instead, she raised an eyebrow. "Some people find them difficult, dear," she said, declining to elaborate on whether these were the people who were about to go off the deep end.

I had more luck with Small's memory strategies, which boiled down to a premise he calls "Look, Snap, Connect." If you take the time to link what you need to remember with a visual image, his theory goes, you'll stand a better chance of encoding and therefore remembering the information. Thus, if you meet a guy named Frank whose last name is Fisher, all you have to do is think of a man fishing, using a frankfurter as bait, and that man's name is yours for life. I tried it at my house when some friends brought their out-of-town relatives to my annual Fourth of July barbecue. Given my troubles with facial recognition, this was a recipe for disaster. How would I introduce this nice couple to fifty friends and relatives in my backyard? Helpfully, the out-of-towners' names were alliterative: Hillary and Howard. To her credit, Hillary was hilarious, and Howard, who happened to be hairless, hung close by her side. Blithely, I introduced Hillary and Howard all evening, "introducking" only slightly by making it necessary for my other guests to produce their own names, which didn't surprise them. I felt like a stellar hostess.

Gary Small advised that by using the same Look-Snap-Connect tactics, I could link several of those visual images, allowing me to remember a boatload of errands. If my Saturday-morning rounds included picking up the dry cleaning, going to the bank and getting some milk, I'd simply build myself a wacky mental picture—perhaps a milk jug dressed in my husband's blue blazer, with a check sticking out of the breast pocket.

There was only one problem, I told Small. I could not recall a time when I'd had a list that short. What about the other items—the soccer tournament, basketball tryout, team snacks, new boxer shorts, dinner reservations, deodorant, sunblock, snorkel mask, stamps, gas, and birthday gift I'd gone after the Saturday before? Even for him, Small concurred, an image like that would be a challenge. This strategy was probably more useful, he admitted, for someone whose kids were grown and gone. A boomer himself, with a couple of kids at home and a working wife, Small acknowledged that he rarely had the time required to build himself a memorable picture.

Nevertheless, I decided to try it. In preparation for my son's elementary school graduation party, I required a large bag of ice, an assortment of pretzels and chips, a jar of salsa and six avocados. That was straightforward enough. I also needed to take my black slingback heels to the shoemaker in preparation for a trip to New York, and to call my friend Flo, who was in charge of setting up our dinner with college buddies. I considered the possibilities. Apologizing to Flo in advance, I mentally sat her in the backseat of my car, with a bag of ice under her feet. The avocados, she juggled. The plastic container of salsa, she wore like a hat. The shoes, which I miniaturized, dangled like earrings. The chips and pretzels were giving me trouble until I took them out of their bags and turned them into a sweater—a little bit over the top, but definitely something you could wear to dinner in TriBeCa. I carried this image with me to the supermarket and the shoemaker, pulling off the errands without a hitch. I even remembered to call Flo. This was great, l thought. I could make up silly pictures and never need a shopping list again. But I think I encoded the information too well. As far as I'm concerned, Flo is still in the back of my car with her feet on the bag of ice. I've never been able to replace her with anyone else—with, say, my brother, who still requires a call back. It seems that Flo, chic in pretzels and potato chips, will occupy the backseat of my car in perpetuity.

There are endless mnemonic strategies, most of which have been employed since ancient times, but my husband revealed one that is indisputably modern. Growing up in New York City, he memorized the numbers emblazoned on the jerseys of New York athletes of the 1960s and 1970s; if you ask him to remember a phone number, he will oblige by summoning to memory the players associated with that particular combination of digits. In order to remember 458883, he'll stand wide receivers Homer Jones, Aaron Thomas and George Sauer Jr. next to each other in his mind. "Of course, you have to remember the players that you choose," he admits. "It helps to have some sort of rationale." He uses this system to memorize phone numbers, street addresses and locker combinations, but it is apparently no help to him when it comes to remembering that the second Tuesday of every month, I'm off to my book group.

"Controlled studies in the laboratory clearly show that ordinary people can use imagery mnemonics to boost memory for a list of words, names and other material," writes Daniel Schacter in *The Seven Sins of Memory*. "There is a problem, however. Many of the imagery techniques are complex, require considerable cognitive resources to implement and are therefore difficult to use spontaneously. The first few times you generate bizarre mental pictures and stories to encode new information, the process may be challenging and fun. But the task of repeatedly generating memorable images can eventually become burdensome enough so that people stop engaging in it."

USING ALL FIVE SENSES

The late Lawrence Katz, a professor of neurobiology at Duke University, who sadly passed away after I interviewed him in 2004, shared Schacter's skepticism about the value of mnemonics and other "tricks" that promise to improve your memory. In his book *Keep Your Brain Alive*, he took a different approach. "I looked through all the books on memory," he explained, "and they all focused on the same thing— learn the rules for mnemonics. The thing is, I can't remember those rules. They involve very complex associations."

Memory and attention are suffering, Katz believed, because sometime in the last couple of decades, we've ceased to engage several of our senses. The world has gone flat, brought to us through a computer monitor or a TV screen. "All television and movies are now designed to activate your attentional mechanism," he remarked. "People are developing a kind of massive attentional disorder, because this stimulation keys into the coarse triggers of your brain. I call it the pornographying of sensation. It makes real life seem pale and timid by association, and we quit paying attention. When it's constant, your brain habituates to it and shuts it off. And imagine, if it has shut out all the loud, dramatic stuff, how easy it is for it to ignore smaller things.

"There are no smells," he announced. "You don't know what anything feels like or tastes like. It's all visual now. Think of a supermarket. Nothing has an odor. We don't like odors. You're supposed to choose your fish or your chicken based solely on the visuals. You're not even supposed to pick up the vegetables to squeeze and sniff them. That's frowned upon. So you miss things like texture, smell and heft. We've become sensorily deprived. It has to do with the ubiquity of visual images—on the Internet, on television, in the movies. We're so saturated with visual images, we quit paying attention to how things smell or sound or feel."

Humans were not intended to go about their lives using just their eyes and ears, Katz explained. "These are inadequate tools for encoding and processing everything properly. The demands on two senses alone are just too great." Katz's approach, which I liked, was to forget the mnemonics and the brainteasers, and to make a concerted effort to restore the sensory experience to your everyday life. You could do this by shopping at farmers' markets, where the "sniff and touch" approach was okay. You could work in your garden, enjoying the sensory bombardment of rich soil and decaying plant material. You could go hog wild, rolling the car windows all the way down on a summer's night instead of immediately turning on the AC. You could make your own spaghetti sauce instead of doctoring up the one that comes in the jar.

In his book, Katz recommends that you try approaching your front door with your eyes closed, or better, while blindfolded. I was reluctant: I'd probably trip over a bagful of baseball bats, or the sneakers that are always left languishing like Pekingese on the doormat. But one morning, just for kicks, after everyone but the dogs had left for school or work, I gave it a shot. Hoping that none of the neighbors were watching this routine, I tied a bandanna over my eyes before getting out of the car. Tentatively, I slipped from the driver's seat to the asphalt driveway, which was a bigger drop than I'd anticipated. I shuffled a few steps to the bump that marked the edge of the grass, found the paving stones and minced my way toward the gate. Unlatching it, something I do several times a day, was quite difficult: Before I succeeded, I stuck my hand in a thick spiderweb. I slid through the opening, tried to refasten the latch so the dogs wouldn't get out, and gave up after several tries. After a brief entanglement with a rosebush, I found the stone step that marked the beginning of the patio, and made my way to the front door. Fishing my bulky key ring out of my purse, I tried to recall the shape and texture of the correct key. Before I could insert it into the lock, I had to kneel and run my hand along the smooth edge of the door until I found the metal doorplate, and then the keyhole. It took another minute to get the right key into the lock, open the door and trip over the threshold, which I'd forgotten existed. I was sure I'd built myself a passel of new synaptic connections, junctions where information is passed from one neuron to another. "The world is really the best brain gym," Katz assured me when I reported my results. "Real activities in the real world stimulate you in ways that no simulated activity can possibly accomplish."

After I told him about my predilection for forgetting the printer paper, Katz gave me another tip, which proved immensely useful. "When you're packing up your stuff for the day, preparing to head out to the office," he said, "don't just say to yourself, 'Hmm, I need printer paper.' Feel that paper. Imagine the weight of it on your arm, those sharp corners, the crispness of the wrapping. And with that paper in hand, envision yourself getting into your car." I followed his instructions, imagining the weight of the ream inside my brown leather tote and the way the straps felt on my shoulder. I envisioned my phone, often left on the kitchen counter, comfortably nestled in the front pocket of my purse. I considered the weight (and smell) of the bag of tennis clothes my son needed for his clinic after school. And miraculously, I remembered them all.

A WAY TO ENHANCE BRAIN PLASTICITY

Although Web-based memory-improvement programs are proliferating, I was reluctant to consider them. I spend all day sitting in front of a computer monitor, and I couldn't imagine what sort of content could lure me to stay longer. Michael Merzenich, a professor at the Keck Center for Integrated Neurosciences at the University of California, San Francisco, who has a reputation for ingenuity (he invented the cochlear implant, an electronic device surgically implanted in the ear that restores partial hearing to the deaf), told me he'd developed a program called HiFi that exercises the brain's auditory and language systems, treating the underlying causes of cognitive decline, rather than just the symptoms.

His work is based on the concept of brain plasticity: Throughout life, the brain remains an organ with a capacity for physical and functional change. The brain has about 100 billion neurons, each of which makes an average 1,000 connections with other neurons, totaling some 100 trillion connections. Plasticity reflects the brain's ability to reorganize itself by forming new neural connections, explained Randy Buckner, a neuroscientist at Howard Hughes Medical Institute. "This reorganization takes place by mechanisms such as axonal sprouting, in which undamaged axons grow new nerve endings and form new connections with other nerve cells, creating new neuronal pathways, thus enhancing learning."

Clusters of neurons, with their extensive synaptic connections, are not restricted to a particular function. If, as a result of aging, one region of the brain—say, the right frontal lobe—isn't working especially well, neurons from a disparate region may be recruited to pick up the slack. Sometimes this happens automatically, but more often, repurposing neurons for new roles requires training. Nor is the human brain limited to whatever neurons were handed out at birth. The existing troops are continuously reinforced. Throughout the life span, new neurons are born and integrated into existing circuitry, in a process called neurogenesis. (The understanding that neurons are able to reproduce is just a decade old; previously, these cells were believed incapable of any form of regeneration.) Increased mental and physical exercise, as well as social interaction, stimulates neurogenesis, especially in the crescent-shaped hippocampus, which regulates many aspects of learning and memory.

"Here's why you lose your memory in midlife," Merzenich said as we huddled in a UCSF meeting room the size of a closet. "It's not because of a true loss of intellect—you're just as smart as you ever were. It's because the quality of the signal is poor. It's like listening to the news on the radio when you're driving through a canyon; the information is all there, but the static is so bad that you just can't get it."

The problem with most memory-training programs, Merzenich said, is that you need an intact memory to use them, and an intact frontal lobe to apply what you learn. You also need a working pair of ears. An uncorrected hearing loss is often a factor in what appears to be forgetfulness. Older adults with mild-to-moderate hearing impairment may expend so much cognitive energy on hearing accurately that they have fewer resources remaining for encoding the material, and thus do not remember *what* they heard. They are experiencing presbycusis, an age-related deficit that occurs when the cochlea—a snail-shaped structure in the inner ear that transforms sound waves into electrical energy—is damaged over time.

People give up on programs that rely on their failing faculties because they feel like they aren't getting anywhere. The tasks are simply too hard. Posit Science's program avoids all that, Merzenich explained, by starting slow and automatically bumping up the level of difficulty when you are able to produce the correct answer at least 80 percent of the time. Posit scientists are working on programs for healthy aging in five broad areas: auditory processing (listening and communication), visual processing (seeing), executive function and associative processing (problem solving), motor control (hand movement) and vestibular processing (balance). The Brain Fitness Program currently focuses on listening and communication. The software costs $495.

"Here's what we don't do," he said. "We don't train people to practice remembering. That's like kicking a dead horse. When you're encoding in a faulty way, it's really not useful to tell you to work harder. I hate all the compensatory strategies that are out there—the 'So what if you can't remember, just write it down' school of thought. That's the road to a continuous decline of confidence."

Merzenich, who in addition to his professorship is also the chief scientific officer of Posit Science, the company that is developing HiFi, noted that they'd tested the program on almost one hundred adults ranging in age from sixty-three to ninety-four, for a period of eight weeks. The participants who completed the program improved ten or more years in neurocognitive status.

For any age group, I acknowledged, that was a huge leap. Would it work as well for people in midlife? Merzenich reported that he'd just put a fifty-two-year-old retired CEO through this training. "He'd made a lot of money," he said. "He'd kicked back for a few years. When he came to me, he said, 'Mike, I feel like I'm slipping. I'm not confident.' We got him down here, gave him the neuropsych battery, and found that he was in the eighty-fifth percentile for his age, which, given his background, was lower than you'd expect. We trained him. By the end of the program, he'd moved up more than a standard deviation—now he's in the ninety-eighth percentile. Six weeks after he finished, he was the CEO of a new start-up. And we do take credit for that, because almost certainly, there was an impact beyond what the test could measure."

HiFi relies heavily on animation. It looks a great deal like *Sesame Street,* only the characters are older folks. (I finally figured out why: Lloyd Morrisett, one of the creators of *Sesame Street,* is on Posit's board of directors.) Each hour-long session involves identifying tones, matching word sounds, and enjoying cartoon characters, mostly quirky senior citizens, who presumably are meant to distract you from the unpleasant matter at hand—listening, at least at first, to ascending and descending auditory tones. I was strikingly bad at the game called Hi or Low, where users decide if tones are rising or falling. Was that tweety-bird sound heading up or down? Most of the time, I couldn't tell. There were other games as well: an audio form of Concentration, where you must find the right match for a sound, and

Sound Replay, where you reconstruct a sequence of syllables that start slow but become much faster. The pace was dreadfully slow—each training session seemed to go on forever. Quickly, I became bored and irritated by the silliness on the screen before me.

With Michael Merzenich at the helm and $23 million in venture capital behind it, this program was the crème de la crème. I'd heard some of my older neighbors talking about it, including one who was a Scrabble champion many times over. It was catching on fast with people in their seventies and eighties, but I thought it was too time-consuming and precious to appeal to people in middle age. I asked about that: Was Merzenich thinking about the huge midlife market? The company was working on a new Web-based program for middle-aged people. It would be possible to download individual exercises, like songs from iTunes, and run them anywhere—for instance, in a hotel room in Japan. I suggested programming the exercises for the gym: Couldn't Posit Science build something that would run on the touch screen of a stationary bicycle?

BREAKING YOUR OWN RECORD

In the end, it was all about attitude. We'd never be attracted to any brain training activity that made us feel old.

An article posted on Slate sent me straight to a Web site called MyBrainTrainer. Bruce Friedman, a fifty-four-year-old Los Angeles entrepreneur had succeeded where everybody else had failed—as president of MyBrainTrainer, he'd "skewed young," as the marketing people say, determined to attract not only boomers, but members of Gen X (the eldest of whom were forty-five), and much younger people headed for graduate, law or medical school. There was nothing on the site to make me feel like I was over the hill or deficient: This was about making still sharp people even sharper. Somehow, MBT (as it is called by those who love it) makes you feel young and hip, no matter how poorly you are performing.

Friedman referred to MyBrainTrainer as "the first mind gymnasium." Appropriately, it includes a Nautilus circuit of nine types of brain exercises, to be performed at lightning speed. The exercises measure reflexes, perception, mental-processing agility, analytical skills, concentration, visual recognition, memory capacity and vocabulary. All of them are short, fast and challenging, and there are innumerable ways to analyze your results. Friedman is into statistics, obviously the kind of guy who gets pleasure from rattling off racing odds or batting averages, and he brought that sensibility to bear on the Web site. All Web-based memory-training programs give you the opportunity to try to beat your last score, but Friedman, who knew the power of the competitive urge, designed MyBrainTrainer so that not only could you compete against yourself, you could run circles around members of your age group or others in your profession. The $9.95 membership allows you to rack up results for four months, by which time the dedicated are so hooked that they wouldn't dream of quitting.

At my request, Friedman introduced me to one of MBT's aficionados, Bill McGlynn, a forty-three-year-old emergency room paramedic technician, who had been using MyBrainTrainer for two years. "I had the sense that my mind was slowing down," said McGlynn in an e-mail, "and I didn't like it. I suspected that I was dealing with some degree of attention deficit disorder. I could be very creative and productive and innovative, but I could also lose focus and fail to pay attention to the details." Lack of focus in normal life was annoying, Glynn explained, but in an emergency room setting, it was dangerous.

After two years of working with MyBrainTrainer, McGlynn was sure that his concentration had improved. "It's great to see progress," he said, "because it makes it easier for me to accept errors I make in the course of the day without becoming overly self-critical." Knowing that his scores were rising, he could silence the voice that asked, "Where will this end?" There was no reason to think, he realized, that he was headed downhill. "I can actually see that I am competent in most areas," he explained, and "in those that continue to be challenging, I'm making progress." Working with MyBrainTrainer makes it easier for him to absorb new medical technologies, which increases his value as an employee, he said.

He cautioned that playing MBT could be addictive. "At first, I put in a lot of time, one to two hours a night, five to seven days a week," he explained. After two months, he cut back to a half hour most days, and eventually reduced his playing time to three fifteen-minute sessions per week. After his infant daughter was born, he tried playing one-handed while he was holding her. "I even tried using my toes," he admitted, "but that was a bust."

In recent months, he'd restricted his playing to coffee breaks at work. Between emergencies, he takes on the MBT Challenge, consisting of seven consecutive games he can play in a quarter of an hour. "In a way," he wrote, "it's a sacrifice, since I work in a very stressful environment. But I find that playing increases my adrenaline level and relaxes me at the same time. The instant measurement—knowing where I stand at that exact minute—really keeps me going. It's very reinforcing."

I tried MyBrainTrainer, and for once, the news was good. I liked it—a lot. It suited me perfectly—the moment of competition in the middle of a busy day, the neuronal boost that made me feel like I'd taken a coffee break. My performance was dependably terrible—my reaction time made a tortoise look speedy. And yet, there was hope. I could feel it. And I could see it, every time my score crept up a point, or even two.

There were other products on the way. Nintendo, the Japanese game company, understood the size of their target market when they launched Brain Age: Train Your Brain in Minutes a Day, to be played on the portable Nintendo DS. At $20 apiece (plus, of course, the $200 outlay for the Nintendo DS system on which to play it), the game proved so popular with aging Japanese baby boomers that the company sold five million of them and quickly released another title, Big Brain Academy. According to Nintendo's marketing materials, the games were designed by a Japanese neuroscientist whose image bobs unnervingly on various screens as he delivers strange translations of what are apparently Japanese proverbs. I suspect that these games are more hype than help. For one thing, your success with the touch screen relies on how well the DS can decipher your handwriting with a Palm Pilot–style stylus and the ease with which the built-in speech recognition system interprets your answers. Brain Age's training focuses almost entirely on processing speed. On the first go-round, almost everybody receives the unsettling news that his brain is at least a couple of decades older than he is. Nintendo knows, however, that boomers like instant gratification. If, with practice, you can scrawl the answers to twenty simple math problems in the blink of an eye, or rapidly memorize and write out a long list of words, suspiciously easy remediation is at hand. After a few training sessions, you'll get the good news: Your brain is now younger than you are. I'm not sure how accurate Brain Age is—my guess is that it's far too limited in scope to know what it's talking about. But it's quick and handy, and I can see the benefit of tackling a few exercises when I'm stuck waiting in some mind-numbing line at the post office.

With MBT, I'd found Intervention #3 and a way to get my sleepy brain to kick over the traces, if only for a few minutes at a time. In my mind, a new question surfaced: What was going on upstairs that made those middle-aged neurons so weary? I rolled my eyes skyward, trying to imagine the structural and biochemical nature of my brain.

8

BATHING IN BATTERY ACID

. . .

Elevated Cortisol Associated with Chronic Stress
Is No Friend to Your Hippocampus

You already know that most midlife cognitive problems arise from deficits in working memory and attention. But "real" memory loss—the failure to hang on to the information that you're positive your frontal lobes have sucked up like a sponge—may also occur in middle age. "Sometimes I pay the closest attention possible," said Jeanette, a research scientist. "I really focus, and I give it plenty of time to register, and still, I don't recall it." When this happens, it's brought about by a glitch in a stressed-out hippocampus, a region of the brain central to learning and memory.

Your hippocampus is situated more or less behind your ears, deep within the temporal lobe of the brain. It is a sensitive thing, with a major role in remembering daily events and information. It is a framer, a setter-in-context, letting you know what happened first and what happened next. It locates you in time and place, constantly updating your coordinates. When Sean, the IT guy, lost his way in his hometown, it's likely that he experienced a hippocampal failure. The hippocampus is a key structure for conscious and voluntary recollection of previously learned information.

Stress is not always bad for your memory; in fact, a little stress in the environment makes your recall sharper. An occasional burst of stress can be neuroprotective—it's like a housekeeping service, sweeping up and disposing of misfolded proteins and other cellular garbage.

The way your body responds to whatever life dishes out—the "stress response system"—will determine whether your hippocampus remains robust or starts to shrivel like a peach in the sun. We talk a lot about "being stressed," but in truth, getting stuck on the crosstown bus on the way to your dental appointment doesn't qualify. To meet the scientific definition of stress, the source must be unpredicted, unpredictable, novel and beyond an individual's control. It can be personal—a sudden death in the family—or environmental, like an earthquake. It can be global and all-encompassing—9/11 and subsequent acts of terrorism fit that description.

It would be fine if stress were short-lived—if, as Stanford neuroscientist Robert Sapolsky described it, you experienced " . . . about three minutes of screaming terror as you sprint for your life on the savanna, after which it's either over with or you're over with." Instead, we live in a chronically heightened state of alertness and anxiety, steeped in the feeling that danger could strike at any time, without warning. Whether or not we're in immediate peril, the brain makes a judgment call and turns on the taps. Then, it forgets to turn them off. "The human mind is so powerful, the connections between perception and physiological response so strong, that we can set off the fight-or-flight response just by imagining ourselves in a threatening situation," observed Bruce McEwen, a neuroendocrinologist at Rockefeller University.

THE PHYSIOLOGY OF STRESS

When your body kicks into overdrive and stays there for weeks, months or even years, your hippocampus suffers. The stress response reflects the body's effort to keep things balanced—to achieve just the right level of oxygen, glucose, acidity and temperature. This process begins in the amygdala, a small almond-shaped structure deep within the center of the brain, where it is connected to other regions, including the hippocampus, through long, myelin-coated axonal fibers. When the amygdala gets the message that you ought to be afraid—whether of your supervisor's expected tirade or your child's midterm grades—it activates the HPA axis, a round-robin involving the hypothalamus, the pituitary and the adrenal glands. There's a volley of hormones, resulting in the release of the first blast of adrenaline, which heightens alertness and sharpens memory.

After a few moments, the adrenal glands ship out a second wave of stress hormones, known as glucocorticoids. In humans, the relevant glucocorticoid is cortisol, a steroid hormone made from cholesterol. To provide fuel for the coming exertion—the fight-or-flight response—cortisol converts into glucose whatever carbohydrates have been stored as glycogen, and sends them roaring into your circulatory system, shipping as much glucose and oxygen as possible to the heart and other muscles. A half hour or so after the stress response is initiated, the HPA axis is supposed to receive a message from the beleaguered hippocampus that everything is copacetic—it's time to shut down the works. If the hippocampus is too impaired to send the message, the "all hands on deck" response continues, and the real trouble starts. Cortisol doesn't allow glucose to do its work very well. It prevents insulin from entering the cell. Thus, people with very high production of cortisol often develop a prediabetic condition called insulin resistance, or glucose intolerance.

Even a few days of elevated cortisol levels can harm hippocampal neurons. (Other hormones in the body decline with age, but not cortisol—there's always more than enough of it to go around.) In rats, observed Bruce McEwen, three weeks of repeated stress (in the rats' case, minor limitations on mobility in their cages) caused cells in the hippocampus to shrink and change shape. The dendrites that normally stick out all around the neuronal cell bodies, like leafy foliage on a tree, grew sparse. The synapses at the tips of the dendrites began to dry up, which meant fewer synaptic connections and a reduced opportunity for information to be transmitted, resulting in mild to moderate memory impairment. High levels of cortisol also result in a sharp decline in the formation of new brain cells. Scientists hypothesize that chronically high levels of cortisol may clamp down on the production of brain-derived neurotropic factor (BDNF), which acts as a sort of fertilizer for dendritic branches and new cells. Without this compound that encourages nerve cells to grow and make new connections, the hippocampus quickly runs out of replacement troops for dying cells and synapses. When neurons atrophy or die in large numbers, the hippocampus itself begins to shrink, severely impairing cognitive processing.

The production of BDNF is controlled by a particular gene. Unfortunately, about a third of the population has inherited a wimpy variant of the gene that causes BDNF to clump inside a cell body instead of being transported to the synapse, resulting in a less luxuriant—and therefore less capable—network. When you say you inherited your father's lousy memory, this could be what you're talking about.

Studies have shown that once the stress response is shut down, BDNF production resumes, and nerve-cell regeneration begins to flourish once again. "The atrophy is reversible," said Bruce McEwen, "when the stress is short-lived. But stress lasting months or years can kill hippocampal neurons."

THE RELATIONSHIP BETWEEN MEMORY IMPAIRMENT AND DEPRESSION

When a patient complains of memory deficits, physicians and psychologists immediately suspect that clinical depression is the catalyst. It's a reasonable assumption—if you're immersed in a gray cloud of melancholy, your preoccupied frame of mind will surely impede your ability to pay attention to what's going on around you. In truth, the association is far more complex. New research makes it clear that no matter what your psychologist thinks, depression alone doesn't cause memory impairment. One hypothesis suggests that the cycle starts with elevated cortisol, which creates stress-induced inhibition of BDNF and restricts the birth of new nerve cells as well as the growth of dendrites and axons, eventually sending the brain into the neuronal equivalent of a midair stall. The hippocampus suffers, and the condition we know as clinical depression surfaces. The longer depression lasts, the more likely there is to be hippocampal shrinkage. In patients who have been seriously depressed for years, the volume of the hippocampus is 10 to 20 percent smaller than in well-matched control subjects. Interestingly, essential fatty acids can go a long way to counteract the cortisol-induced reduction of neurogenesis. Scientists have observed that depression is sixty times rarer in countries such as Taiwan and Japan, where people consume a lot of oily fish, compared to the United States and Germany, where fish is infrequently on the table.

The more I thought about it, the less surprised I was that hippocampal injury could generate symptoms of clinical depression. If the function of the hippocampus is impaired, it makes it impossible to set life events in context, to frame them in terms of significance. How easy it becomes to fall into an existential fog. The hippocampus tells you who you are, and why you are. A reduction in its function could obliterate your sense of self.

New research suggests that hippocampal injury accumulates with recurrent depressive episodes, and if the depression is untreated or treated too late, some features of cognitive impairment will persist. Prompt treatment with antidepressants appears to offer protection to the hippocampus. Antidepressants that inhibit serotonin reuptake, such as Zoloft and Prozac, stimulate the brain to get back in the business of producing BDNF. (Although invaluable in the treatment of major depressive disorders, antidepressant medications are by no means benign. Taking these medications, especially for extended periods, can result in various types of cognitive impairment, a state of affairs I'll describe in further detail in Chapter 15.) "The reason that SSRIs require about a month to begin to alleviate the symptoms of depression," said Fred Gage, whose team at the Salk Institute for Biological Studies in La Jolla, California, discovered the ongoing nature of neurogenesis, "is that it takes that long for newly born cells . . . to fully mature, extend their dendrites and integrate with existing brain circuitry." This observation puts to rest the highly speculative idea that SSRIs work by increasing the level of serotonin in the brain. It is likely that new approaches to the treatment of depression will involve drugs that intervene much earlier in the cycle, perhaps by reprogramming the HPA axis and scaling back on the production of cortisol before it can do so much damage to the hippocampus. Investigators are considering the potential of drugs that manipulate cortisol levels. Eventually, these pharmaceuticals may replace antidepressants for the treatment of many mood disorders.

Post-traumatic stress disorder presents a significant threat to the hippocampus, and therefore to memory. It affects 8 percent of people at some time in their lives. Symptoms include intrusive memories, nightmares, flashbacks, an increased startle response and heightened vigilance, social impairment and problems with memory and concentration. "Post-traumatic stress disorder patients have their fear alarms essentially 'turned on' at all times, so they don't have the ability to make the fine distinctions that will help them determine when a true threat enters their environment," noted J. Douglas Bremner, director of the Positron Emission Tomography Center at Emory University. In PTSD, soaring levels of cortisol damage hippocampal cells over time, and the hippocampus shrinks, causing cognitive impairment. In a neuropsychological study of patients with PTSD, Bremner found that their scores on a group of tests were, on average, 40 percent lower than normal.

ARE YOU STRESS PRONE?

"Stress proneness," as Robert S. Wilson and his colleagues at Rush University Medical Center in Chicago refer to the trait, is not a promising sign. In a study of nearly eight hundred people in their seventies, Wilson and his colleagues found that people prone to distress experienced a tenfold decline in their ability to recall events in their lives. In this group, comprising elderly Catholic nuns, priests and brothers, people who were highly prone to stress (in the ninetieth percentile) demonstrated double the risk of developing Alzheimer's disease than those with a lower degree of vulnerability to stress. Even those who did not develop Alzheimer's disease showed considerably more memory impairment than subjects with low-stress ratings. Although the details remain fuzzy, scientists theorize that there is a connection between chronic stress, depression and the development of Alzheimer's disease. Hippocampal cells left defenseless by the continual onslaught of cortisol may be particularly sensitive to the encroachment of the protein aggregates that eventually become amyloid plaques.

In my days as a mom-around-the-playground, I observed firsthand the varying thresholds of stress in small children. Some melted down at the first sign of truck-snatching. Others took the slide face-first, sucked gravel, dusted themselves off and went on, bleeding slightly, to play another game. I'd noticed the same discrepancy in adults: Some sprouted tendrils of anxiety at the least provocation, until they became as rigid and choked with it as a pot-bound asparagus fern. Others let most things roll off their backs—nothing was too big a deal. Without exception, the asparagus ferns—that sensitive, stress-prone group of which I was a card-carrying member—complained of more serious memory deficits than the easygoing types.

A few dozen survey respondents explained that as far back as they could remember, they'd been vulnerable to anxiety; it was as if their threshold was set too low. Things that didn't faze other people set them on edge. They wondered if they were born that way. It was possible, I told them. A Columbia University study of stressed or depressed mothers and their unborn babies showed that when the expectant mother was presented with a stress-inducing computer task, the stress response showed up in the fetus. Jerome Kagan, the child development expert at Harvard, noted that by the age of sixteen weeks, infants placed in unfamiliar environments show either uncomfortably high sensitivity for new stimulus or calm interest in exploring it. Remarkably, that response at four months of age is a fairly accurate predictor of how bold or timid that infant will be as an adolescent or an adult.

EARLY STRESS RESULTS IN MEMORY DEFICITS IN MIDDLE AGE

I was skimming through the fat packet of scientific-journal research articles that my researcher sent me on the first of every month when a headline grabbed my attention: "Early Life Psychological Stress Can Lead to Memory Loss and Cognitive Decline in Middle Age." The study explored the relationship of rat pups and their mothers. Tallie Baram, a professor of anatomy and neurobiology at the University of California, Irvine, limited the nesting materials in crates inhabited by newborn pups and their mothers. Rats require plenty of fresh straw and cotton to be comfortable, explained Baram, and limiting this resource made motherhood stressful.

Initially, the pups appeared to do well enough. For some months, through adolescence and young adulthood, they were indistinguishable in behavior from other rats. Then something changed. As the group approached what qualifies as middle age for a rat, they began to show signs of memory lapses. In their maze tests, they forgot locations and objects they had seen the previous day. As they continued to age, their memory deficits grew worse, and developed at a much faster rate than rats raised for the first week of their lives in an environment where nesting material was plentiful.

The problem, Baram found, emerged from deep in the brain. The cells of the hippocampus, the crescent-shaped region responsible for processing, storing and recalling new information, were not firing properly because synaptic connections had deteriorated and the numbers of synapses had dwindled.

The hippocampal network (so called because it consists of several interconnected components) functions something like the childhood game of Mousetrap. In that game, you drop a small silver ball in a tiny plastic bucket and watch it make an elaborate circuit, rolling down chutes and bumping over stairs, until it accomplishes the course and triggers the trap. In the brain, information from the frontal lobes zips down myelin-coated axons to the hippocampus, where it jumps from synapse to synapse, making its way from the subiculum to the dentate gyrus. Eventually, it circles back to the subiculum, where it is consolidated. At that point, ready for long-term storage, the information is shipped back to the frontal lobes, where (under ideal circumstances) it becomes a matter of permanent record.

Tallie Baram's investigation was groundbreaking because it revealed that early life stress damaged the hippocampal network in a way that would not become apparent until middle age. The exact nature of the association remained unclear: Was that bedding shortage simply a metaphor for another kind of deprivation? Baram hypothesized that the paucity of soft cotton and straw sent the mother rats into crisis mode, altering the way they raised their offspring. Baram's research suggests that a subtle alteration in the relationship of rat mother and pup was enough to reprogram the expression of specific genes, and send the HPA axis into chronic overdrive, over time causing injury to the hippocampus.

(People talk, all the time, about their "good genes" or "bad genes," supposing, incorrectly, that hereditary genetic disposition is as immutable as a cameo brooch, passed down through generations. Although some genes code physical characteristics like eye color, the majority of genes offer only a suggestion and environment influences the rest. Environment plays a role in determining which genes will be switched on—"expressed"—and which will be turned off. There are specific genes that influence the function of the HPA axis, which regulates the stress response.)

Michael Meaney, a professor of psychiatry at McGill University, shed more light on this theme. In his "licking behavior" rat study, he spelled out the precise cascade of molecular steps by which early environmental factors program gene expression, and thus regulate the pups' lifelong stress response.

Like human mothers, rats have different nurturing styles—some mothers lick and groom their pups three to five times more than others and make it easy for them to nurse, while others are more aloof. The two styles are equally effective from an evolutionary perspective: Rat pups survive and reproduce at the same rate. Meaney split his rat population into two groups, according to mothering style. He found that the pups of frequent lickers were more exploratory in new surroundings, less fearful, and less reactive to stressors as adults.

The pups of frequent lickers also remembered things better. Their main task involved swimming through a floating labyrinth to search for submerged objects. The offspring of frequent lickers outperformed their peers, learning spatial relationships faster. They retained what they learned longer than their less-licked counterparts. When researchers analyzed their brains, they found that the well-nurtured rats' hippocampi contained more synapses. The pups of enthusiastic lickers also had higher hippocampal concentrations of the neural receptor that tells the body the stress response has been sufficient and it is time to shut down the flood of hormones, suggesting that the gene that orders up the amino acids that eventually build neural receptors was fully engaged. The more care a pup received, the lower the level of the stress hormones in the bloodstream.

Although in terms of our genetic makeup, rats and humans are very similar—rats and humans share about 90 percent of their working DNA and all of the same disease genes—it is always risky to make the leap from rodents to humans. The former, for one thing, are born blind, and are totally reliant on touch, while human infants are subject to much broader influences. Still, social scientists latched on to Meaney's and Baram's studies, suggesting that emotional stress associated with parental loss, abuse and neglect in childhood resulted in memory deficits in middle age. The implications were fascinating, though insufficiently explored. If early deprivation could begin the cascade of stress response, elevated cortisol levels and hippocampal damage, perhaps it was possible, through intervention, to find and hit the switch that would turn it off.

THE ROLE OF PARENT-CHILD ATTACHMENT

When I developed the survey at the beginning of my research, it never occurred to me to ask about people's childhoods. Nevertheless, many volunteered the data. It seemed that the more disturbed an individual's childhood had been, the more apt he or she was to experience cognitive problems in adulthood. Those whose lives were unquestionably stressful in the present, but who had grown up in secure, nurturing circumstances remarked that "stress made them sharper," or "helped them get things done." Those who had emerged from a rockier environment observed that they were "decked by stress," "became really stupid and out of it under pressure," and "found it harder and harder to deal with the total blank I tend to draw when I'm under fire."

Those who had experienced stress early in their lives often reported that they had trouble with context—what came first and what came next. They had only the vaguest recollections of their early years, but more recent events in their lives were also foggy. Their mental mapping and spatial skills were weak. These were all hippocampal functions, not to be confused with the failures of attention that reflect changes in the frontal lobes. There were exceptions, of course, but in general, the more challenging the circumstances of birth and early childhood, the more impaired hippocampal functions appeared to be.

"It would not be an exaggeration," wrote Anna, a sculptor, "to say that I have almost no memory of my childhood. There's nothing at all before the age of ten, and just scraps after that. I can't see myself in my own memories—at best, they are like individual frames from a Super 8 movie, tiny glimpses of who I was. There is nothing full-blown about them, no emotional content. I am very barely there."

In every case, I found, there had been a significant roadblock in the relationship between mother and child—mental or physical illness, including alcoholism and depression, or simply a profound ambivalence toward motherhood. My own talented and ambitious mother, born a decade too soon to have understood that she had the option of postponing motherhood or choosing a career over a family, found herself ill-prepared, at the age of twenty-four, for the task of caring for me, a colicky and demanding infant. From remarks she made over the years—and by her astonishment at my enthusiasm for caring for my own babies—I recognized that for her it had been a difficult time. Had it made a difference?

Daniel Siegel, a psychiatrist in private practice, and the director of the Center for Human Development at UCLA, has spent most of his career studying attachment relationships in human mothers and children. He finds that when mothers are emotionally unavailable, imperceptive, rejecting, unresponsive, or disorganized and disoriented in their relationships with their very young children, those offspring grow up to become adults who lack "conceptual anchor points that . . . allow access to memory, including fluidity of narrative and the ability to self-reflect."

I telephoned Siegel, and asked if I could bring two salads up to his West Los Angeles office, just to make sure I had it right. His hypothesis seemed, well . . . anti-mother, to say the least. We sat at a large, round table, gazing at the hills of Brentwood, stretching all the way to Bel Air, through a stretch of window glass.

He estimated that only 55 to 65 percent of infants are blessed with secure attachment. "Attachment relationships," he began, "may serve as the central foundation from which the mind develops. The pattern of brain function is shaped, I believe, by this relationship. When an infant is presented with an unsolvable problem, meaning that the parent who is supposed to protect her is exhibiting frightened, dissociated or disoriented behavior, it's inherently cognitively disorganizing."

"How do you know," I asked him, "when you've got a patient who had an emotionally avoidant or ambivalent mother?"

"The tipoff," he said, "is that this person doesn't recall his or her childhood experience. Life is lived without any sense of the past.

People wind up with a complete lack of recall for the personal events in their lives, particularly in regard to relationship-related experience. Their memories are weak or nonexistent, and the sense of self is not rich."

Emotionally avoidant or ambivalent mothers come in many stripes, but rarely are they physically abusive to their children, observed Siegel, which would require more involvement than they could muster. Often, the avoidant or ambivalent relationship arises from a more complex family situation—the presence of an alcoholic husband, for instance, could make it impossible for a human mother, as distressed as a rat without enough soft bedding, to emotionally attach to her offspring.

"Attachment establishes an interpersonal relationship that helps the immature brain [the child's] use a mature brain [the parent's] to organize its own processes," explained Siegel. Children who do not have the opportunity to take advantage of a mature brain grow up unable to set things in context, always struggling to find a way to jigsaw together the pieces of a life. By the age of ten in these children, Siegel found in his research, "there is a unique paucity in the contents of their spontaneous autobiographical narratives"—the story of their lives, as they grasp them. In infants without the benefit of secure attachment relationships, it is likely that cortisol runs high. The stress response kicks in young, and becomes an inherent part of the child's metabolism, injuring the hippocampus, as it had in Baram's rats. When the hippocampus is robust, Siegel explained, it's a remarkable time machine, allowing you to travel forward and backward through your life. When it is inundated with cortisol, particularly at a young age, the hippocampus fails to provide a sense of consequences, of logical expectations, knowing what comes first and what comes next, and what general form an event ought to take.

"You know," Siegel said gently, "sometimes when people address these attachment struggles, the cognitive problems and the intimacy problems begin to resolve."

I wondered if he'd give me another fifty minutes, starting right then.

9

YEARNING FOR ESTROGEN

. . .

Rejecting Hormone Therapy Could
Leave Your Neurons in the Lurch

Everyone who knows me is convinced that the minute I turned fifty-two, I developed attention deficit disorder," said Peggy, the consultant, who acknowledged that this was unlikely. "I struggle to concentrate, and only the threat of total annihilation helps me to buckle down. I can't remember what I read, or what people tell me." She suspected that menopause might have something to do with it, although hers had "come and gone in about forty-five minutes, with no particular symptoms."

When I told Peggy that her neurons were likely begging for supplementary estrogen, she was shocked. Like a lot of women of menopausal age, she had rejected hormone replacement therapy as too dangerous, and, from everything she read in the magazines, probably unnecessary.

Estrogen's role in the brain is only beginning to get the attention it deserves. Neuroimaging has allowed scientists far more insight into cerebral metabolism. Sufficient levels of the hormone are essential for neurons to properly utilize the neurotransmitter acetylcholine, critical for optimal function of the hippocampus and frontal lobes. Estrogen also increases the rate of neurogenesis and helps neurons build new synaptic and dendritic connections, limiting the damage wrought by an overabundance of midlife cortisol. The hormone has shown a remarkable ability to fight off the ravages of beta-amyloid, the protein that builds the nerve-cell-destroying plaques that accompany the development of Alzheimer's disease. Estrogen also helps protect brain cells against the destructive effects of oxidation, while stimulating glucose metabolism and cerebral blood flow. Recent evidence suggests that it may also slow the shrinkage of gray matter, the darker-colored tissue in the brain that is composed mostly of the bodies of nerve cells that are critical for information processing. When you consider that currently a woman can expect to live nearly one-third of her life in postmenopause, it's hard to overestimate estrogen's importance.

"It's overwhelmingly clear in the literature," said Stanford neuroscientist Robert Sapolsky, "that estrogen is critical in terms of keeping neurons from becoming dysfunctional and dying." The difference in tests of verbal fluency (where women are called upon to name, for instance, as many zoo animals as they can think up), between postmenopausal women who take estrogen and those who do not, is one-half to one standard deviation. That's not a huge gap, but for many women, it's significant enough to be noticeable.

WHI RESULTS ALARM PHYSICIANS

"But didn't that big study a few years ago find that everything about estrogen was dangerous?" Peggy asked, furrowing her brow in concern. She referred to the Women's Health Initiative, a large prospective study of sixteen thousand women, instituted in the early 1990s to assess the benefits and risks of hormone therapy and determine whether long-term combined treatment with Prempro (conjugated estrogens and progesterone) and Premarin (estrogen extracted from mare's urine) could prevent coronary heart disease in women.

Over a period of several years, starting in 2002, the WHI produced nothing but bad news. Different aspects of the drug trials were halted as results reflected a moderately increased risk of breast cancer, stroke and blood clots. The participants showed no reduction in the rate of heart disease, and actually demonstrated a doubled risk of developing dementia.

Understandably, doctors hurried their patients off the drugs. In the first eight months of 2002, before results were generally known, 45.2 million prescriptions were written for HRT. In the same period in 2005, the number declined to 24.7 million. Almost overnight, HRT was transformed from a generally approved treatment to a dangerous therapy of questionable value. If HRT was prescribed at all, the FDA asserted, it ought to be prescribed at the lowest effective dose for the shortest time possible.

For a while, I bought that line of reasoning, as did most of the women I knew. We were coping well enough with perimenopausal symptoms. When the big "M" hit, we'd soldier on, refusing to give in to the hot flashes and the mood swings. "I'm stocking up on a lot of those cute camisoles with the built-in bras," quipped one well-toned acquaintance. "If I have to, I'll strip."

Women who were cut off from the drugs midmenopause were less sanguine. Jill was taking care of her sick mother and a pair of recently adopted six-year-old twins when the WHI results hit. "My physician told me to get off HRT and I did," she said. "Immediately, I could feel my metabolism changing. I had hot flashes daily, and I didn't sleep well for a year and a half. I was totally distracted."

Like many other women, Jill noted that she was having trouble finding words. Her spatial skills had also diminished, leaving her vulnerable to what she called "Vessel Identity Syndrome." Often, she found herself searching her car and house for her lost phone (which she was sure she'd put in her purse), only to find that she'd put it in her briefcase.

She was also affected by What Am I Doing Here? Syndrome, where she'd find herself standing in her bedroom closet, unable to remember what she'd come upstairs to get. Her hippocampus, the region of the brain responsible for orienting her in place and time and determining context, was likely suffering from estrogen deprivation.

"For me, it was like day and night," said Lucy, the retail marketing director. "One day, I was fine. I barely needed a calendar. And then I was bombarded with all sorts of perimenopausal symptoms, the worst of which involved memory and concentration. It got so bad that I was having trouble doing my job. I couldn't remember what anyone had told me, or what I had read. I had awful problems with people's names, even people who had reported to me for months." One woman, an esteemed professor of cognitive neuroscience, remarked: "I really felt like my memory was shot. The change was so scary to me that I thought I'd better get myself evaluated. But of course, I knew everybody in town who would be qualified to evaluate me. So I figured I'd have to find someone in a city about an hour away. Before I did anything about it, my friends started commenting on the same deficits, and I thought, 'Thank God, maybe it isn't pathological.'"

Jane Gross, writing in the *New York Times,* tried to wean herself off HRT shortly after the WHI study was published. She mourned her loss. "Ask any woman who has had a difficult menopause if she thinks that Mrs. Rochester, locked in the attic in *Jane Eyre* was actually insane. The answer is likely to be a resounding 'no.' Poor Mrs. Rochester, living in an era before hormone therapy, has been on my mind lately as I have tried, unsuccessfully, to wean myself off estrogen. Like me, she was probably dazed from too many sleepless nights, frightened by palpitations with no apparent cause and unable to concentrate on the simplest task or read a sentence from start to finish."

The cognitive problems often accompany hot flashes, although sometimes they arrive alone. One woman, a sales executive, reported that the day before, she'd asked her assistant to arrange a 9:00 A.M. meeting of the entire staff. Attendance was mandatory. When she arrived in the conference room, a minute or two late, she looked around at a dozen sleepy faces and realized that she'd forgotten what the meeting was about. "I was so humiliated," she writes. "I could feel the heat rising, the pores opening. I explained that I needed some more information and raced back to my office. As soon as I looked at my desk, I knew what it was that I wanted to talk about."

I noticed that some women long entrenched in successful careers were hitting fifty and quitting. No doubt, some had simply had enough of the daily grind. But others seemed to be feeling the cognitive squeeze. At the local Starbucks, I ran into the executive who supervised four hundred people, the one who had told me the year before that her memory remained impeccable. She'd declined to renew her contract, she said. She'd had enough. As we were leaving, she stopped in her tracks, looking deeply confused. "Um, I don't seem to have my banana bread," she said. I pointed to the Starbucks bag swinging from her elbow. She clapped a hand to her forehead and looked downcast.

GIVING THE PROPER TESTS

Gayatri Devi, a neurologist who has long studied estrogen's utility in the brain, runs the New York Memory Clinic. She often sees professional women of menopausal age who suspect that they are in the early stages of Alzheimer's disease. "I get them all the time," she told me in a phone interview. "Editors of magazines, people who run multinational companies—very high-powered individuals, almost always in their midforties to early fifties. What's happening to them freaks them out at a level where they definitely do not need to be freaked out. They're in the boardroom, and suddenly they just cannot find the right words, or they have no idea of what has been said. It's alarming. It's humiliating, at a time when their careers are really peaking. These women are accustomed to functioning like sports cars—they expect to go from zero to sixty in six seconds, and then, unpredictably, it takes them a minute. Or sometimes, they can't accelerate at all. When we test these women, we see that they score at a very high percentile in language and verbal skills, but working memory is very weak."

In past generations, notes Devi, this midlife change in cognitive abilities might not have been as troublesome. "The kinds of skills required of a middle-aged woman at home—making dinner, keeping house, tending grandkids—after menopause, these remain intact. What starts to go are abilities that require very rapid thinking—the skills you need in the workplace. The irony of it is that the more mentally agile you've been in your life and career, the less you've trained yourself to rely on supports and struts. Those who always had excellent memories, who could cite you chapter and verse, never had to be very organized, because their brains could handle the demands. When that agility is no longer there, the infrastructure collapses."

Many research studies have shown that supplementary estrogen, given after menopause, improves cognitive function. But what remains ill-defined is what happens to brain function during the years immediately before menopause, known as perimenopause. The results of several investigations of women in this stage, who received neuropsychological tests, showed that specific types of memory remained perfectly intact, and in some cases improved. That was confusing until a team of researchers from the University of Rochester Medical Center rounded up twenty-four perimenopausal women who complained of memory problems, and put them through a battery of neuropsychological tests. They concluded that the women were not imagining things: There were clear deficits in their ability to encode new information.

Gavatri Devi wasn't in the least surprised. Her patients are usually given a full neuropsych battery, which often reveals striking deficits. "For years," she said, "I've known that researchers were giving the wrong tests, usually the MMSE, which is far too easy. In order to see the effect of disappearing estrogen, you have to give women tests that tax them to their limits. And you have to test the skills that are affected."

WITH ESTROGEN, AGE MATTERS

"To be honest," said Grace, a nurse-practitioner, "those WHI results scared the pants off me. As soon as I read them, I called up every menopausal or perimenopausal woman I know, and even some older women who I thought might still be taking HRT, and told them they should call their doctors and make plans to get off."

At the time, her reaction seemed prudent. Like millions of health care providers across the country and around the world, Grace did not have a complete grasp of the scope of the Women's Health Initiative study.

The sixteen thousand women who were recruited for the WHI study were, on average, 63.5 years old, more than a decade older than the women who usually take HRT. As I mentioned, the intention of the trial was to assess whether Wyeth Pharmaceutical's hormone replacement therapies provided long-term protection against the development of cardiovascular disease. An ancillary trial called WHIMS (the MS stands for Memory Study) examined the hypothesis that HRT could help prevent Alzheimer's disease. The women enlisted in WHIMS were even older, between the ages of sixty-five and seventy-nine. (The investigators chose women substantially beyond the age of menopause, reasoning that they'd get their results more quickly than they could if they had to wait for a younger group of participants to grow old.)

Wyeth had been lobbying for many years to have the FDA extend the labeling on its HRT drugs to include information about the drugs' ability to prevent heart disease. The results, Wyeth expected, would extend the market share, solidifying HRT as a treatment that women began taking to alleviate the symptoms of menopause and stuck with for years. Without a large clinical trial, the FDA refused to approve the drug for prevention of heart disease, and so the WHI study was born, funded in large part by the drug company, which had little doubt about the investigation's outcome.

Frankly, I wouldn't have wanted to be in Wyeth's boardroom when the results started coming in. A scientist who was present told me the shock was palpable—absolutely no one in the company had expected to see these unfavorable findings. As scientific trials go, this was the gold standard, a very large, prospective, double-blind, placebo-controlled study. It took months for the investigators to figure it out.

As I've mentioned, the women selected to participate in WHI and the ancillary study, WHIMS, were well past menopause, and a great deal older than those who usually take HRT. At the start of the study, more than half were being treated for hypertension, 11 percent were diabetic and over a fifth were obese. They were at high risk of cardiovascular and cerebrovascular disease, which in turn would influence their cognitive functioning regardless of hormonal treatment. Although the results of WHI were startling, it seemed unlikely that they would generalize to younger women who initiated HRT at menopause.

Over time, scientists realized that age was a crucial factor in the success of hormone therapy. Researchers hypothesized that there was a "window of opportunity"—a critical period in a woman's life when estrogen was neuroprotective. This window opened, they suggested, in the late forties, around the time of perimenopause, and closed a year or two after loss of ovarian function. They conjectured that if estrogen treatment was initiated too late—well after menopause—instead of being protective, it might well be deleterious and exacerbate mental deterioration. The late introduction of estrogen appeared to inhibit the production of BDNF, once again stalling neurogenesis.

There's a distinct possibility that the WHI study results have at least as much to do with the toxic effects of the synthetic progesterone in Prempro as they do with the administration of estrogen. Three decades ago, when research revealed that hormone therapy with estrogen alone caused uterine tumors in postmenopausal women who had not received hysterectomies, doctors added progesterone—primarily Prempro—to the cocktail, making hormone replacement therapy a great deal safer. Unfortunately, Prempro has its own side effects. It can be sedating, have a negative effect on mood and reduce the activity of the neurotransmitter acetylcholine. In a study at Rice University, postmenopausal women who used both progesterone and estrogen performed far worse on cognitive tests than those who used estrogen alone.

ARE SYNTHETIC ESTROGENS THE ANSWER?

Researchers are working on developing estrogens that don't need to be balanced with progesterone or can be used cyclically with smaller amounts of progesterone, thus limiting an individual's exposure. There are two types of estrogens—alpha, which engenders feminine characteristics, found in breast, cardiac and uterine tissue, and beta, which targets brain and bone. Scientists are working to devise "designer" estrogens that will function selectively, leaving the heart, breasts and uterus alone, while providing protection to neurons and bone cells.

Roberta Diaz Brinton, a professor at the USC School of Pharmacy, and her colleague Liqin Zhao are at the forefront of this research. Their new formulations are neuroSERMS—selective estrogen receptor modulators that target and activate estrogen mechanisms in the brain, while avoiding estrogen receptors elsewhere. Their plan is to develop drugs that easily penetrate the blood-brain barrier, promoting cognitive function while preventing age-associated neurodegeneration in both men and women. So far, Brinton's lab has produced 32 molecules that meet the criteria, plucked out of a field of 532 candidates. "To work properly," noted Zhao, "a neuroSERM would have to behave as an estrogen, promoting the growth of dendritic spines and encouraging the development of new synapses in the regions of the brain involved in memory function. It would also have to activate neuronal defense mechanisms, as estrogen does, when confronted with a damaging agent, like beta-amyloid."

Because neuroSERMs lack the feminizing effects of the synthetic estrogens currently produced by pharmaceutical companies, they may eventually prove useful for both men and women. Although the mechanism remains ill-defined, like their female counterparts, male neurons also have an affinity for estrogen, which in men is converted from testosterone to a form of estrogen called estradiol.

Indeed in both genders, the development of Alzheimer's disease may be closely linked to the level of estrogen present in the brain. One study, published in 2005, reported that women who died with Alzheimer's had much lower levels of estrogen in their brains, and a greater load of amyloid plaques than age- and gender-matched control subjects. Men who develop Alzheimer's disease generally have half the level of available testosterone of men who remain healthy. Whether the protective effect derives from testosterone itself or from testosterone that has been converted to estradiol remains to be studied.

PATIENTS RETURN TO HORMONE THERAPY

Many of the physicians who ordered their patients off HRT suggested that they try so-called natural hormones, bioidentical compounds usually made of yams and soybeans, but also formulated from herbs such as black cohosh. In the wake of the WHI study, spending on menopause remedies shot up, topping $100 million. Because it contains estrogenic compounds, soy is considered unsafe for women with family histories of estrogen-dependent cancer. Although the administration of soy may result in the reduction of other menopausal symptoms, the results of two clinical trials reported in the *Journal of the American Medical Association* show that soy isoflavones are not effective in preventing menopause-associated cognitive decline. Nor is black cohosh guaranteed to be what the label says it is: In recent tests at Columbia University, three out of eleven samples of the herb were adulterated, and clearly misbranded, in violation of federal labeling regulations.

As physicians become more aware of the unrealistic parameters of the Women's Health Initiative study, their patients with debilitating hot flashes, insomnia and mood swings are beginning to return to hormone therapy. (Note that the *R,* standing for "replacement," has been dropped from the acronym, an FDA move that reflects the agency's more conservative stance.) "I tried all the other stuff," writes Lucy, who quit HRT as soon as the WHI study was published. "The black cohosh, the red clover, the soy—but my hot flashes and insomnia were killing me and my memory loss and inability to concentrate were getting worse. Now that I'm back on it—this time I'm using the estrogen patch—I feel a lot more like my old premenopausal self. I'm much clearer in thought and action. I think it's a personal choice, like all your choices about your body."

Over the early months of 2006, I watched the health experts back away from the notion that hormone therapy was to be avoided. A new wave of studies appeared, reporting results that make it clear that timing is everything. Data from the Nurses' Health Study showed that women who went without estrogen for a long period after menopause were more likely to develop atherosclerosis, the clogging, narrowing and hardening of the bodies' large arteries and medium-size blood vessels, which limits blood flow to the brain, weakening neurons, and can also lead to stroke and heart attack.

Hormone therapy continues to be contraindicated for women who are predisposed to breast cancer, blood clots, heart disease or strokes. The rest of us are free to take it or leave it. If, like Lucy and Jill, we choose to take it, we may do it at least as much to benefit our brains and arteries as to alleviate our hot flashes.

For me, on the cusp of fifty, the window of opportunity was just opening, and I had a choice to make.

10

THE VULNERABLE BRAIN
· · ·
The Repercussions of Concussions
You Never Knew You Had

It took a while, but I finally received a copy of the results of the neuropsychological evaluation I'd had at UCLA. I already knew that my diagnosis was "normal, age-consistent memory impairment," but as soon as I opened the envelope, I realized that this wasn't as straightforward as it had seemed. A few of my scores, in tests of verbal proficiency, were very high. Others—five, to be exact—fell into the category marked "below peers." I wondered—okay, I'll admit that I obsessed—over what that might mean. How exactly was it that I had come to inhabit the bottom of the heap?

Irritably, I called Gary Small to ask him how he could have possibly described my performance as "falling within normal range." It was simple enough, he explained. My high and low scores knocked each other out. When they were averaged, I fell right in the middle, which made me a viable participant for the 14-Day Memory Prescription Program research protocol. There was, he pointed out, a distinction between "falling within normal range" and *being* normal. "You have to understand the difference between a research protocol and a clinical evaluation," he said. "It's not the same as going to a private physician."

Frankly, I hadn't understood that: I thought I'd learn at UCLA everything there was to know about my condition. As it turned out, that wasn't in the cards. Given the dramatic skew in my neuropsych results, Small suggested that it made sense for me to have a clinical evaluation with a psychologist who specialized in tracking down the underpinnings of cognitive impairment. "It might help you understand your strengths and weaknesses, so you can continue to function at your peak," he said. I stopped grilling him for answers, and decided to look elsewhere.

A FULL NEUROPSYCHOLOGICAL BATTERY

A few days after that conversation, I received a call from a gentleman who had recently sat beside me at a dinner party. One of his colleagues, a neuropsychologist, was studying high-achieving people who develop cognitive problems in middle age and later in life. I told him to go ahead and give him my number.

Soon after, Jonathan Canick phoned. He was a clinical neuropsychologist, he explained, with a subspecialty of evaluating and assessing intelligent people whose deficits were rarely identified with typical cognitive tests. Over the years, he'd customized a battery of tests that could tease out the subtleties of dysfunction. He'd Googled me, so he knew where I'd gone to college and most of what I'd been up to professionally for the last twenty-five years. At his request, I read off my UCLA results, including the three scores in the "very superior" column and the five scores in the "below peers" column. On these tests, he explained, for most adults, the difference in skill level between individual tests is somewhere around 10 percent—between half a standard deviation and a full deviation. As it stood, I was crossing more than three standard deviations. To put it mildly, that was unusual. He questioned whether what I was experiencing was a consequence of normal aging.

"But I fall within normal limits," I reminded him. "It says so right here."

Without bothering to mince words, he told me what he thought of Small's protocol, and his tests. "You have gone through what was presumably a very thorough evaluation at UCLA, with the best technology in the world, and as far I can see, they totally missed the boat," he said. "An average score is an average score for an average person," he explained. But for a person who at one time had been superior or very superior, an average score is an indication that something is awry. If Albert Einstein had a twenty-point IQ loss, he explained, he'd continue to perform far better than "normal," but he himself would feel the difference. "Many of the areas in which you are struggling don't typically show changes until you reach your sixties or seventies," he said. "It's absolute nonsense to suggest that these are normal age-related impairments. Coming from your academic and professional background, achieving at the level that you have typically achieved, what you are experiencing is far from normal."

I was taken aback, I must admit. I'd grown accustomed to the idea that my cognitive glitches, however irritating, were perfectly average and age appropriate. Now Canick was telling me something different. With trepidation, I faxed him the UCLA results, and made an appointment to go see him the following week at California Pacific Medical Center, where he is chief neuropsychologist. I was well on my way to Intervention #4.

As soon as we sat down, he extracted a sheet of paper from the unfiled mountain on his desk and quickly sketched a bell curve—essentially a large, inverted U. Down the middle, he drew a vertical line. "Anything on or near this line," he told me, "is average." Then he plotted the points of my UCLA scores. A few clustered near the middle. Several were all the way to the right, in the superior range. Then he moved his hand to the far left side of the page—the area where scores below average lie—and there, he made a few more dots. "This last one would actually be off the page," he said, "but for now, we'll put it here, at the edge."

When he finished, he leaned back in his desk chair, stretching his legs. "You are all over the map, from the twenty-fifth percentile to the ninety-fifth. In other words, you demonstrate a combination of impressive competence and incredible deficiency." He suspected there was nothing wrong with my memory, which he defined as my ability to retrieve information that I'd already consolidated. "I'll bet that your memory is dynamite," he said. "Whatever is going on with you is more likely about working memory and attention. If it blows by you and it doesn't register, you're never going to be able to retrieve it, because it doesn't exist."

Over the next two days, for more than seven hours, Canick put me through my cognitive paces. Numbers, letters, words, figures—they kept coming, and there was no time to rest. He wanted to wear me out so that I'd be unable to compensate for my deficits. He was succeeding: As each half hour passed, my performance diminished. "Keep going," he said, when my energy and attention flagged. "Go to the end." He worked my brain like a trainer probing for weakness.

After lunch, he had a stack of papers in his lap, and some preliminary results. When we first spoke on the phone, he acknowledged, he'd believed that my problems arose from a perimenopausal condition. He'd now changed his mind.

"Then what is it?" I asked. "Panic? Anxiety?"

"Not at all," he said. "From what I have seen so far, the panic and anxiety show up only when your brain shuts down. You are suddenly, inexplicably, cut off from all you know, which is surely disturbing."

He went over my scores on the tests he'd given me that morning. He'd shown me a flip book with dozens of black-and-white head shots. Then, after a few minutes, he showed me a similar book with the same pictures plus some additional ones I hadn't seen before. My job was to tell him which faces were familiar. I had no idea: I'd have done just as well if I were blindfolded. Nothing about their faces rang any bells. No wonder I was unable to identify celebrities the rest of

America knew on sight. My performance on a test where I was asked to connect the dots through an ascending lineup of letters and numbers was no better: I lost the sequence and had to backtrack to recover it. Nor was I able to reverse a short string of numbers and repeat it back to him.

Each test told him something about the function of a specific part of my brain. In my case, the frontal lobes and the right temporal lobe were reluctant to get up and go to work. I processed information far more slowly than he'd expected, which suggested that synaptic connections were impeded.

"For now," he said, "it's only a hypothesis, but your symptoms and your test results show the distinct neurobehavioral fingerprint of brain damage, the kind that emerges from a series of mild traumatic brain injuries."

"I don't think so," I said, certain that he was mistaken. "I've never even been knocked unconscious."

HARD ON THE OUTSIDE, SOFT ON THE INSIDE

Canick explained that concussions don't always result in loss of consciousness, or even in amnesia. One can have a mild concussion, experienced as "feeling dazed" or "seeing stars," and still remain conscious. All that is required is rapid acceleration or deceleration of the head. This motion is often accompanied by the rotation of the brain inside the skull, the interior of which is composed of eight cranial bones. The bones in the prefrontal cortex, home to the frontal lobes, are jagged, with sharp protrusions. When the brain, which is the texture of softened butter, makes contact with these protrusions, small blood vessels may rupture. This releases blood in an uncontrolled way into the cranium, which, unlike other parts of the body, cannot expand to encompass it. Microscopic tears develop in the myelin sheath surrounding axonal nerve fibers, which release their lipids, followed by swelling and the formation of scar tissue. The real damage shows up weeks or months later, often after the injury has been forgotten, as ruptured axons begin to die, carrying fewer and fewer impulses, reducing the capacity to process information efficiently.

Because this process occurs on a molecular rather than a cellular or structural level, it is invisible to PET and MRI. Newer technology—in particular, diffusion tensor imaging, which measures the ease with which water molecules move in a particular direction through axons—can trace axon fiber tracts in the brain and detect structural abnormalities in specific neural pathways. But so far, that technology is restricted to experimental applications. I'd have to take Canick's word for what had happened.

Even if a first injury did little harm, Canick explained, the second injury could have an exponentially greater impact. "Second impact" syndrome is common among athletes and often results in a dangerous increase in pressure inside the skull, which can cause permanent damage.

NEW IDEAS ABOUT MILD TRAUMATIC BRAIN INJURY

Until a decade ago, scientists regarded mild traumatic brain injury—where patients do not lose consciousness and there is no structural damage—as inconsequential. Patients were expected to recover quickly and entirely, and anyone who presented symptoms after a month or two was considered to be "malingering," probably in the interest of settling a large lawsuit. Extensive research, mostly on rodents, at the University of Pennsylvania's Head Injury Center, revealed the fallacy of this assumption. Not only could a mild traumatic brain injury result in cognitive deficits that surface after months or years, researchers found that repetitive mild brain trauma accelerates the emergence of Alzheimer's disease by increasing free radical damage (free radicals are attracted to the sudden bounty of lipids released from myelin on sheared axons). It also stepped up the formation of amyloid plaques, hastening the death of hippocampal neurons. (A study published in 2005 reported that retired National Football League players face a 36 percent higher risk of developing Alzheimer's disease than other males the same age.)

I'd smacked my head quite often in my life, I'd told Canick. I always wore protective headgear, but I was active, and there were horseback-riding accidents, ice-skating rack-ups, and biking collisions, all of which left me temporarily dazed. I assumed this was the normal consequence of the shock of taking a tumble. I'd survived years of aggressive downhill skiing without any broken bones, but after many falls I'd seen stars as I lay in the snow, preparing for the arduous job of collecting my belongings from all over the hill. Then there was the matter of my coordination: I am five feet ten inches tall, and like a perpetually gangly teenager, I don't have a good grip on where I end and the rest of the world begins. Low-hanging lintels (the horizontal supports above doorways) and tree limbs positioned just above eye level have caught me in the forehead time after time.

When I was about nine, I was playing in the basement when my younger brother, a whirling towheaded kid drunk on centripetal force, decided it would be fun to spin in circles, an old broomstick extended horizontally from his hands. I was in the wrong place. The impact knocked me flat. For the next three weeks, my eye sockets and forehead turned every color in the rainbow. When I remembered this incident, I grabbed the broom out of the closet and headed for the driveway. I began to spin, faster and faster. I've never taken physics, but even acknowledging that my longer arms, which increased the radius, would be a factor in determining the velocity of travel, it seemed that when my younger forehead met that broomstick, the impact must have been immense. Thinking back to the years after that accident, I remembered debilitating headaches, deemed psychosomatic, which left me pale, damp and nauseous. I also recalled a series of nosebleeds, not the "tip your head back and here's a Kleenex" variety that occasionally strike my children, but great, gushing fountains of blood that flowed for no apparent reason and were difficult to stop. I came upon a study that suggested that in young children, blows to the forehead can have long-term repercussions: Growth in the brain's frontal regions continues through young adulthood, and early injury there can damage formation of the protective myelin insulation and neurons.

I had not, I admitted to Jonathan Canick, taken exceptionally good care of my head. I figured that as long as I wore a helmet, I was safe. What was inside could take care of itself.

He explained that mild traumatic brain injury was much more common than most people thought. According to the National Center for Injury Prevention and Control, at least 1.1 million people each year sustain MTBIs, as they are known. That number is no doubt too low, Canick said, because most people who sustain such "minor" injuries do not go to the emergency room or a doctor's office. They go home and lie on the sofa with a bag of ice on their heads, and when the egg-shaped swelling goes down, they figure that they're perfectly okay. It was impossible to say how many middle-aged adults who presumed they were suffering from age-related memory impairment were actually feeling the consequence of a series of earlier head injuries.

A BAG OF ICE WON'T FIX IT

It was a sobering thought, the vulnerability of the head, how often we injure it—and how little attention we pay. In the course of a year, my elder son fell backward off his skateboard, banging his head. He dribbled trickily in reverse, smack into the post that supported the basketball hoop, knocking himself flat on his back. He'd miscalculated and ridden his bicycle (helmeted, of course) headlong into the partially raised garage door. That was just for starters. Each time, I got out the bag of frozen peas we kept handy for such injuries. He wasn't unconscious. He wasn't vomiting, or particularly sleepy. Like every mother I knew, I figured that meant he was okay.

Adults were by no means off the hook: One fall work weekend, up at an isolated Tahoe cabin, I left my scraping and sanding task to go outside for a minute—where I found a fiftyish man I didn't know lying on the ground at the base of a twenty-five-foot ladder, blinking, confused and rubbing his head. He wasn't sure how long he'd been there. "Hey, I'm fine," he told me as he staggered to his feet. A few months later, on a family trip to a dude ranch, I stood waiting for my horse with a family of four—two young daughters, mom and dad—all of whom wore Stetson hats. When I asked why their heads weren't more suitably protected, I got an earful. Helmets might be okay for lily-livered Easterners, the father explained, but he and his family were from Idaho. Five minutes later, I watched his wife lose her balance when her horse spooked, sending her tumbling to the ground. There was an awful sound when her head met a railroad tie at the side of the trail. When they brought the truck around to take her to the hospital, she was still unconscious. Several days later, I saw the father and his daughters in the ranch lounge. How was his wife? She'd be okay, he said—she was still in the hospital, conscious, but shaken up and bruised. It was a heck of a thing to happen on a vacation, but his girls had been out riding every day—and they still weren't wearing helmets.

Alexa, a travel-company owner, reported that while on vacation, she visited an art gallery, and was just ambling along, reading an artist's brochure, when she walked directly into the low-hanging horizontal branch of a baobab tree and knocked herself flat. More recently, she was cleaning up a Coke that had exploded in the little refrigerator under a granite countertop in her family room. She stood up suddenly, and wham—she was down again. When I told her the stats on head injury, she was shocked. She had no idea that her cognitive problems might emerge from these repetitive traumas.

Other people let me know that minor accidents had changed the course of their lives. Peter, a geophysicist with many scientific publications on his CV, reported that he'd been waiting in his car for a traffic light to change when he was hit from behind by a teenage driver. "She wasn't going more than five miles an hour," he said, " and the impact wasn't much. I didn't bang my head on the windshield or anything." The damage to his car was minimal, but not so the damage to his brain. Within a few months, he'd been overtaken by cognitive deficits. He could not hold multiple thoughts in his head, nor did he have enough memory to execute the complex calculations that are an integral part of his work. "I lose track," he said. "I don't know where I left off." There were problems with reading and speaking as well. He'd been unemployed for over a year.

Trisha, an arts administrator, recounted the details of another automobile accident. Late on a Saturday night, her boyfriend, who was driving her home from a dinner party, barely avoided another car that plowed through an intersection. The couple's vehicle spun around, grazing several parked cars, but when they came to a halt, they were amazed that they'd escaped without a scratch. The next day, Trisha developed a severe migraine headache. It took three more weeks for her to realize that her memory and attention were noticeably impaired. "It was a huge change," she said. "Like everybody else, I'd experienced the typical age-related stuff—forgetting people's names and movie titles. This was very different. Many times a day, I'd put something down and two seconds later, I couldn't remember where I'd put it. I'd agree to meet a friend, and forget about it before I got a chance to write it down. I'd sit down to do some work, and in ten minutes, I'd experience fatigue like I'd never known in my life."

TESTS THAT MAKE YOU WANT TO CRY

On my second day of testing, Jonathan Canick pulled out the big guns. He asked me to name all the words I could think of that started with the letter C. After twenty words that came really fast, the well was empty, and I was stumped. (There are, by the way, a great many obscenities that begin with the letter C. I thought of every one of them, but used none.) "You started out in the ninety-ninth percentile," Canick told me, "and ended up in the first percentile." He explained that what I'd experienced was very common to people with brain injury. It was called "proactive inhibition." Under pressure, instead of continuing to work, the brain shuts down.

Further testing revealed that although my verbal comprehension was very strong, my working memory, the process that allows you to hold several thoughts in mind simultaneously and manipulate them, was significantly impaired. My visuospatial skills were downright pathetic.

I was nearly weeping by the time I finished the PASAT, the Paced Audio Serial Addition Test, a gut-wrenching trial that theoretically separates the brain-injured from those who are simply mathematically incompetent. At first, the challenge seemed simple enough. A recorded voice presents sixty-one single digits, at three-second intervals. The job is to add two consecutive digits, give the sum, forget about it, return to the second digit you'd added and add that one to the next digit down the line. I found myself shouting the number I'd need to add, whispering the sum, and trying to keep all systems online. I sounded like a lunatic. The numbers kept coming, until eventually I broke down.

"I'm lost," I said. "I'll just sit here until it's over."

Canick explained that an undamaged brain takes a few seconds to figure out the pattern, and then runs with it, showing consistent improvement as the task progresses. I started out okay, at twice the average for someone of similar age and education, but by the end, my score was in the highly impaired range.

"It's a very clear metaphor for who you are," he said. "You're two people, one of whom is very smart, the other of whom is, at best, average. You're constantly on an elevator ride between the two levels, and you honestly can't predict how you'll perform on any particular cognitive task. There is a gross, disproportionate falloff as cognitive demand increases and you can retrieve less and less."

"I don't want to be two people," I said

"Hey, that's the good news," said Canick. "Because if you were just one person, you'd be hopelessly impaired. As it stands, you can leverage your intelligence and existing ability in service of the deficit."

I hoped so, I told him. But how?

Head injuries make a person much more vulnerable to mental fatigue, he told me. "You have to put a lot more effort into things that were effortless before. That which was once automatic must now be manual. Your capacity for complex attention—where there's a lot of stuff involved in a single task—or divided attention, where you must split your focus—is very limited. As soon as we tax your attention, you drop two or three standard deviations."

Was he sure—absolutely positive—that what I experienced didn't emerge from stress or anxiety?

"If I were you, I'd leave the psychological interpretations out of it," he said. "In fact, I'd consider putting away all notions that your difficulties are rooted there. You've had a series of mild traumatic brain injuries, and it's really no surprise you are where you are."

He had some wise words for me. "Your expectations for yourself are very high," he said. "And you're your own worst enemy when you don't live up to them—the prospect of failure derails you further." There, he definitely had my number. He warned me that several of my favorite life strategies—working very long hours and driving myself relentlessly—would exhaust me, make me less productive, and eventually result in further injury. Mental fatigue would always be a problem. I ought to plan, he said, on needing the help of talented and sensitive assistants for the rest of my career. Along with excellent organizational skills, they'd need to have the ability to read my mind and catch me before I fell off a cognitive cliff.

In the months after I met with Jonathan Canick, I saw the potential for brain injury just about everywhere. My children jibed that I'd probably like them to wear seat belts and helmets while they sat on the family room sofa. I told every parent I saw, especially those whose children played football, about what I'd learned: Sports injuries account for more than 20 percent of the mild traumatic brain injuries each year. Many, if not most, go unrecorded. There's a skate park next to our middle school where lots of kids admire the acrobatics of our local thirteen-year-old trick-bike star. He's a talent, all right, getting ten feet of air, somersaulting and twirling his bike as if it were no more cumbersome than a baton. His parents, I've been told, are both doctors, but his head is bare naked. The other kids, my son included (except when I catch him), tend to wear their helmet straps flapping fashionably loose. I have to think it is only a matter of time before the EMTs pull up and someone's life is changed forever.

According to Jane Brody, writing in the *New York Times*, each season, one high school football player in five suffers a concussion. Most of these are repetitive head injuries, which increase the odds that the player will experience long-term cognitive impairment, resulting from second-impact syndrome. The subtle effects of a concussion cannot be precisely measured in a cursory sideline evaluation. High school athletes recover more slowly than NFL players, showing longer-lasting deficits in tests of reaction time, concentration and memory. A recent study reported that when a high school athlete develops a migraine after a concussion—even a week after a concussion—it means that the brain has not recovered completely, and that he or she is at risk for a repetitive injury. Until recently, few high school team coaches (and virtually no parent coaches of younger athletes) were aware that a player who "had his bell rung" or reported "seeing stars" or feeling dazed must be sidelined, even if he or she seems to have recovered completely and is itching to get back in the game. A computerized battery of neurocognitive tests called IMPACT, devised by Mark Lovell, the director of neuropsychological testing for the NFL and the director of the sports medicine program at the University of Pittsburgh, is now available to high school teams. It allows athletes to take an individual preseason baseline test and store the data to use for comparison throughout the season.

There's very little in the way of research about how to best rehabilitate a patient who suffers from mild traumatic brain injury. A new study, from the University of Cambridge, UK, suggests that the same drugs used to treat the early stages of Alzheimer's disease, known as cholinesterase inhibitors, which increase the availability of the neurotransmitter acetylcholine, may have a role in treating MTBI. Another test that's in development can track cellular debris—fragments of axonal fibers that do not belong in the cerebrospinal fluid of healthy humans—offering an early indication of the severity of damage.

ANOTHER OPTION FOR TREATMENT

When I reconnected with Jonathan Canick, he said that although he'd heard of brain-injured people being treated with cholinesterase inhibitors, he thought I might have more success with the psychostimulant drugs that had worked so well for several of his mildly brain-injured patients. About a year before he evaluated her, one of his patients, a bright, successful woman in her late thirties, was in a serious automobile accident. Afterward, her neuropsych scores hovered in the seventieth percentile. She seemed unlikely to recover further. After a few months of taking stimulants—in her case, Ritalin—he retested her, and her scores improved by nearly a standard deviation, well into the ninetieth percentile.

Although I knew that Ritalin and Adderall were commonly administered to young children who had been diagnosed with ADHD, I was very reluctant. I hated pills, I told Canick. I was acutely sensitive to drugs, and inclined to react in unforeseen ways. I once spent a night in a hospital emergency room, I told him, after taking theophylline, a drug that is commonly prescribed for asthma, but that made my heart beat so hard I thought it would burst from my chest. I imagined myself red-eyed, buzzing all night, a speed-freak mother in the suburbs. Nothing about this appealed to me. Frankly, I didn't like the idea of needing chemically synthesized help to get through my days. I could do it alone, I told myself. Doing it with drugs sounded suspiciously like cheating.

Canick left it up to me. With a stimulant onboard, he said, he'd watched patients who had been stuck for a long time make huge improvements. If I wished, he'd give me a referral to a bright young psychopharmacologist he knew, who would evaluate me and decide whether I was a candidate for this type of therapy. I told him I'd think it over.

11

COSMETIC NEUROLOGY
. . .

The Potential for Pharmaceutical Cognitive
Enhancement Is Vast and Possibly Irresistible

Waiting in the pickup line at the pharmacy, preparing to collect a perfectly legal prescription for speed, I was beset with doubts. A week earlier, I'd consulted with the psychopharmacologist Jonathan Canick had recommended. For an hour, he'd asked me fairly transparent questions about my mood. Had I experienced manic episodes? Had I ever been suicidal? He measured my blood pressure, which as always, was pleasingly low. Did I take any other drugs? Had I ever been addicted to anything? I told him about my program of vitamins and supplements. That was it, I said. I didn't drink coffee, because caffeine sent me into a tailspin. In fact, I thoroughly disliked the effect that most drugs had on me. After minor abdominal surgery, I took a single Percodan, sat around for three hours with my head spinning, and threw the rest in the trash.

The psychopharmacologist agreed with Canick that I was a good candidate for Adderall. It might be just the thing to give my sluggish neurons a lift. Just about anyone who took the drug experienced increased energy and a subjective sense of greater ability. But people with specific frontal-lobe deficits in attention, whether they emerged from ADHD or brain injury, demonstrated objective improvements on neuropsych tests, specifically in the realm of working memory, processing speed, mental mapping, problem solving and organization.

The clerk handed over my Adderall XR (extended release) in a little white bag, into which she had tucked a product-information sheet, warning me that amphetamines, which the FDA has included in its list of Schedule II drugs, have a potential for abuse and that administration of them, for prolonged periods of time, could lead to severe psychological or physical dependence. Once again, I asked myself what on earth I was doing. I thought of all the writers who had pursued their addictions to amphetamines straight to hell—and shuddered. I had Intervention #5 in my hands, and frankly, it scared me.

I reminded myself that I wasn't exactly on the cutting edge here: In 2005, nearly 1.7 million adults ages twenty to sixty-four and 3.3 million children took psychostimulants, including Adderall, to treat ADHD. The number of adults who received treatment with these drugs leapt 19 percent from the year before. I wasn't surprised by the figures. Over many months of research, dozens of people had asked me if there was a pill that would solve their cognitive problems, or if one would become available "before it was too late."

"If there's any such thing," my local optometrist told me, as I admired his array of imported eyeglass frames, "I'd definitely want it." Why? I asked him. What was the need? He had a thriving business, right in the middle of town. People admired his taste and his skill, and it would never occur to me to resent the fact that he didn't recognize my name when I telephoned. "It would relieve so much pressure, so much stress," he said wistfully, "if I could just rely on myself to remember."

In my travels, I'd met several people who told me that they'd been using smart drugs—or cognitive enhancers—for years. One of them was Lawrence Roberts, a sixty-eight-year-old computer engineer who in his youth had been one of the builders of ARPANET, the military technology that led to the invention of the Internet. In his early fifties, he told me, he felt his mind beginning to change in discomfiting ways. "I could hardly handle the engineering tasks that had been simple for me a few years earlier," he said. "My creativity was still flourishing, but I didn't have the memory or attention to do the kind of work I'd done in my thirties and forties." With the blessing of his wife, a physician, he began a program of dietary supplements and vitamins, as well as an every-other-day dose of piracetam, a pharmaceutical commonly used in Europe to boost mental clarity. Heeding the new research on the relationship between testosterone levels and the development of Alzheimer's disease, he took supplementary doses of the hormone. He also took DMAE, a compound that some say increases the production of the neurotransmitter acetylcholine. He used Deprenyl, a drug that some studies suggest helps protect dopamine receptors from experiencing typical age-related decline. He topped off this cocktail with a little Adderall.

"So," I asked, when I visited him at his house in the hills above Palo Alto, "did it help?"

"I just designed a completely new router," he said, "unlike anything that's out there. It's much cheaper and much faster, and it was my work, from concept to completion. It's hard to describe how demanding a project like this is of memory. There's so much to hang on to—in the short term, and over weeks and months, that most guys my age have long since given up. But I just accepted $20 million in venture money to get the thing rolling. So, yes, I'd have to say that what I've been doing works."

TRYING ADDERALL

The morning after I picked up my prescription, I went to my office and shook a two-tone blue capsule into my hand. I observed it warily. I had warned my husband that I'd be playing Jean-Paul Sartre that morning (he took stimulants every day, in order to write), and that he should check in with me in a couple of hours to make sure that I was not jumping out of my skin. I got myself a glass of water and gulped down the pill. The bright young psychopharmacologist had assured me that at such a meager dose—only 10 milligrams, about the same quantity that a pediatrician would prescribe for a ten-year-old child with ADHD—I wouldn't feel a thing. Within fifteen minutes, I knew for a fact that he was mistaken.

I've viewed enough dizzying charts illustrating nerve-cell transmission to have a pretty good idea of the party that was going on in my brain. Because the drug blocks the reuptake of dopamine and norepinephrine and also stimulates the release of dopamine, there are more of these two neurotransmitters than usual kicking around in the gaps between synapses. The receptors on the surfaces of the neurons embrace this bounty, snapping up molecules, opening ion channels, and notifying DNA to issue orders for the manufacture of various proteins, which relay signals to cells farther down the line. The result: an increase in my level of attention and ability to resist distraction, which I appeared to have taken to extremes. Every item in my visual field—the arm of my chair, my tea mug, the big silver power button on my laptop—was suddenly as riveting as if it were the Hope diamond. I felt wildly attentive.

The first few days had some rough moments. At times, I felt like a nervous wreck, and I couldn't imagine how anyone who was such a mess could show an improvement in thinking. By the end of the week, however, I started to see results. The gears in my brain were meshing. There was synthesis. At work, I was going great guns. I found that I could manipulate several streams of information at the same time, moving sentences around in a manuscript without finding myself holding a handful of orphaned words. My domestic life proceeded uneventfully. I could fly through Walgreens in record time and scoop up everything I intended to buy. In places that previously I found intolerable—like Blockbuster and Best Buy—I was able to bear the onslaught of audio and visual stimulation for up to fifteen minutes at a time.

Most happily, I seemed to possess, for the first time in over a decade, some semblance of a mental map. It was the gift, I knew, of the extra dopamine in the frontal lobes. Suddenly, there was an executive in charge of my executive function. The transformation seemed too remarkable to be evidence of the placebo effect, but I took a wait-and-see approach.

I'd kept Jonathan Canick informed of my progress. When he heard the good news, he asked that I come in and take a few more tests. I knew he had high hopes, and I was afraid that I might disappoint him. On a brilliantly sunny afternoon, I returned to his office. Immediately, I noticed that I wasn't as sleepy as the last time I'd been there. In fact, I was a little wired, perched on the edge of my seat, ready for anything he might want to throw at me. First we took on the flip book of head shots, to test my skill at facial recognition. This time, there was no equivocation. In the second go-round, it was as clear as day to me who I had seen before and who was a stranger. This was a strange sensation, something like waking up in the morning and peering in the mirror to discover that you're not at all the person you were when you went to bed.

The next test, where I listened to a series of numbers and repeated them in reverse, a process that places a heavy load on working memory, had destroyed me in the initial round of testing. No such problems this time. I reversed four digits, then five, then six, then seven, then eight. I knew exactly how to do it. I visualized each digit falling into its slot, much in the way that racehorses enter the gate. Then I took on my favorite task: naming as many words as I could that started with the letter C. Suddenly, my vocabulary was larger. Canick was poker-faced, but I was giggling.

When we moved on to mathematical word problems, I found that I had enough working memory to retain the identity of numbers and objects—six doughnuts, four apples, three bananas, and their respective owners, Jim, Joan and John—long enough to produce correct answers. I longed to return to fifth grade, so I could show off. My frontal lobes were finally doing their job, after a very long hiatus.

At the end of the session, Canick informed me that on the test of facial recognition, my scores improved from far below average—in the nineteenth percentile—to the ninety-third percentile. On the test where I repeated the digits in reverse, I'd made a similar leap, moving from the fiftieth percentile to the ninetieth percentile for people my age. Canick was beaming: These were exactly the results he'd hoped to obtain. "I think you will continue to improve," he said, "as you use this success to build other successes."

I gave him a big hug and thanked him for restoring my memory. "There was never anything wrong with your memory," he reminded me. "What has improved is your attention and concentration, which allows you to manage multiple streams of incoming data."

The story might have ended there, my salvation found in a vial of two-tone blue capsules. But something nagged at me. After a month on Adderall, as my recovered cognitive skills began to feel less like a new party dress and more like a dependable pair of sneakers, I noticed that my daily existence left something to be desired. I worked like a demon, but found myself disconnected from what I'd describe as ordinary human requirements. I was never hungry, which might have been a plus for someone who wanted to lose a few pounds, but I was wasting away. I found that certain pleasures, like wandering around aimlessly in my own mind, were no longer available to me. I was on, all the time. I phoned Edward Hallowell, the psychiatrist who specializes in ADHD (and who has the disorder himself), to find out whether many of his patients experienced these disconcerting feelings.

He acknowledged that some did, and often it was a matter of adjusting the dosage. I asked him if he took the drugs himself. "Oh, God, no," he said. "Stimulants make me hypervigilant. I just take coffee." The fact that he prescribed them widely but avoided them himself I found mildly ironic.

I began to take minivacations from Adderall—a Sunday off so that I could recline in a lounge chair and watch my kids perform crazy clown dives at the local pool. Slowly, I began to suspect that I was gunning a middle-aged engine at speeds better suited to one with fewer miles on it, and that there would be consequences. Because I'd never experienced the feeling of euphoria that causes some people to desire ever increasing levels of the drugs, I wasn't concerned about becoming addicted. I was, however, worried about psychological dependence. When the Adderall wore off, around 5:00 P.M. each day, my mood plunged. I was exhausted, tense and often grouchy. My children informed me that I had misplaced my sense of humor, that the mother they preferred had been replaced by a robotic go-getter.

As it turned out, my personality hadn't changed. By the end of the day, I was, unfortunately, in drug rebound. Having acclimated to extra snacks of dopamine and norepinephrine, my brain grew sullen when forced to function without them. There was some sketchy research suggesting that eventually, this situation might become permanent. My dopamine receptors could become desensitized to normal levels of the neurotransmitter, which would further impair frontal-lobe function. There were other reasons not to take psychostimulants: In 2006, an FDA advisory panel of drug-safety specialists found that the drugs were potentially more dangerous to the heart than Vioxx or Bextra, two pharmaceuticals that had been withdrawn from the market in recent years.

EXPLORING OTHER OPTIONS

I wondered if there was a safer, less exhausting way to improve my attention. I'd read several studies that reported promising results from an alertness-promoting drug called modafinil, manufactured in the United States by Cephalon under the brand name of Provigil. In 1998, the FDA had approved Provigil for the treatment of narcolepsy, a genetic disorder of the nervous system that scientists believe emerges when certain proteins, called orexins, produced by a small number of nerve cells in the hypothalamus, are destroyed as part of an autoimmune reaction. Narcoleptics find the desire to sleep irresistible. Even when they are not extremely sleep deprived, they drop off every chance they get, which makes it impossible for them to hold most jobs, or, for that matter, to drive a car. In 2004, the FDA also green-lighted Provigil for the treatment of excessive daytime sleepiness, related to such conditions as obstructive sleep apnea and shift-work disorder. Unlike Adderall and Ritalin, Schedule II drugs that come with all kinds of warnings about abuse, Provigil was a Schedule IV drug, which meant that there was no indication that its use resulted in dependence or addiction. Scientists had determined that unlike Adderall and other psychostimulants, Provigil did not rely on dopaminergic pathways to do its work.

They knew what it didn't do—but no one, including Jeffry Vaught, who runs research and development at Cephalon, could identify exactly how Provigil enhanced alertness. "That's really not so unusual," said Vaught. "There are plenty of drugs where the exact mechanism of action is not understood—for instance, lithium and acetaminophen." He didn't seem in the least unhappy about this gap in Provigil's labeling. If no one could figure it out, this would allow Cephalon to maintain its lead in a vast and mostly untapped market. When I ran several scientists' explanations for Provigil's efficacy by Vaught, he chuckled. "People say they know how it works," he said. "I guarantee that they do not."

In a way, taking Provigil isn't very different from drinking coffee—if your caffeine intake could be calibrated, so that you got the ideal amount all day long. "There are two systems for arousal," explained Vaught, "working in discrete regions of the brain. One of them—the one Provigil targets—is highly selective, promoting calm, attentive wakefulness. The other system—the one caffeine, cocaine and amphetamines target—comes along with a lot of baggage, which is why people lose their appetites, have trouble sleeping and find themselves feeling on edge." With Provigil, Vaught said, there is no edge. There's no euphoria, either, which reduces concerns about drug dependence. Nor is there evidence of a withdrawal syndrome. You can take Provigil when you need it, and stop on a dime.

A study from the University of Cambridge, UK, by Barbara Sahakian and Danielle Turner, both of whom are at the leading edge of research on cognitive enhancement, determined that in healthy volunteers, modafinil (the generic name for Provigil) induced reliable improvements in working memory. The scientists had their subjects perform a test called the one-touch Tower of London planning task. This involved moving stacking colored doughnuts from one configuration into a different configuration, in a specific number of moves. When the subjects took modafinil, they suddenly found the drug improved planning, decision making and verbal and visual memory—essentially, every cognitive skill we need to get through the day.

The drug also seemed to cut down on impulsivity. "People are more reflective," said Turner, "and less likely to leap before they look, which increases the chance that whatever answer they are going to make is correct." At the root of impulsivity is the brain's inability to inhibit behavior—to get a grip on the reins and pull up short. Distraction is one manifestation of impulsivity, reflecting the brain's inability to restrain itself from dividing attention. It was not unreasonable to think that Provigil could put a stop to the kind of cognitive lollygagging that plagues so many of us.

When I returned to the psychopharmacologist for my monthly check-in, I told him I'd had enough of Adderall. I'd done the research, and I was convinced that Provigil was worth a try. Unfortunately, he'd never heard of it. Neither had Jonathan Canick. Because of its very specific indications—for narcolepsy and daytime sleepiness—pharmaceutical reps never mentioned it to mental health professionals. It was usually prescribed by a neurologist or a sleep-medicine specialist. Once again, it was time to move on.

I sent Anthony Chen, a research fellow in cognitive neuroscience and neurologic rehabilitation at the University of California, San Francisco, my neuropsych report in advance of my first appointment. When we sat down together, he'd read it from start to finish, which was no small feat—it was thirty-seven single-spaced pages long. I told him that my brain had worked much better on Adderall, but that I didn't like the side effects. It might be a matter of changing the dose, he said, but since I was already at the bare minimum of 10 milligrams, he suspected that I just couldn't tolerate stimulants.

There were alternatives, he said. I waited for him to bring up Provigil, but he didn't. Like several doctors before him, he pointed out that my insomnia was likely responsible for my memory problems. It was something I'd have to fix. I was waiting for the inevitable discussion of sleeping pills, which came and went mercifully quickly. I pointed out that the idea was to improve my cognition, rather than impairing it further with sedatives, which in my experience engendered overwhelming brain fog.

Instead, he strongly recommended that I try a program of mindfulness-based stress-reduction therapy, essentially a meditation class that focused on relaxation and left out the spiritual component. He also thought that the time had come for me to have an overnight sleep study, where every aspect of my sleep physiology would be identified through polysomnography. I could do it at Stanford University, which has an excellent sleep-medicine program.

I was willing, I said, to try both of these approaches. In fact, I'd already made inquiries at Stanford. Then, I started talking about Provigil. I told Chen that everything I'd read about it in the scientific journals suggested it would improve working memory and attention, which from Jonathan Canick's neuropsych report, he could see represented the lion's share of my problem. The drug would eliminate my daytime sleepiness, which suggested that I might sleep straight through the night. If Chen was disconcerted by the onslaught of information, he didn't show it.

He agreed that the drug might well work for me. Before I could try it, I'd have to get off Adderall, and stay off for a full month. He reminded me that I needed to wean myself off Adderall slowly, or risk suffering symptoms of withdrawal.

As it turned out, even though I carefully tapered the dosage, getting off Adderall was no picnic. I gritted my teeth through the first week while my brain bellowed for dopamine and norephinephrine. In retribution, it behaved like an overtired child in a supermarket cart, petulantly tossing items overboard. I suffered from Colliding Planets Syndrome, as unreconciled requirements from various aspects of my professional and personal life smashed into each other at high speed. One day, I missed the frying pan completely and dropped a freshly cracked egg—which would have hit the floor, if it hadn't landed on my little black dog, providing a bonanza for the larger yellow one. If there was any consolation, it was that there were better days ahead.

Once the Adderall was out of my system, I noticed that I felt more intuitive and creative. Was it possible, I wondered, that drugs like Adderall and Provigil that inhibit impulsivity also clamp down on the aspect of cognition that allows ideas to meld in unexpected and marvelous ways? For those who relied on logical, one-foot-in-front-of-the-other thought, such restrictions could be helpful. But what about people like me, for whom impulsivity—the sudden, irresistible mental leap—paid the bills? What would have been lost if Leonardo da Vinci, a man who undeniably suffered from a deficit of attention, had been able to get a grip on his free-associating brain?

Five weeks later, I took my prescription for Provigil to the pharmacy, ready to give it a try. The pharmacist scowled as he peered through his reading glasses. They didn't carry it, he said, and it would take at least a week to get it in stock. Seven days later, I presented myself at the pickup window and took the brown vial of white, oblong pills home.

Provigil and I got off to a rocky start. I swallowed what for most people would be an extremely conservative dose—100 milligrams, half of what's prescribed for narcolepsy—but within a half hour, I felt far too wired, as if I'd had ten cups of coffee. The next morning, I got it right. All I needed was half a tablet, just 50 milligrams of Provigil, taken around 10:00 A.M., after my brain knocked out a few hours of work and started to sputter and smoke like an engine that had run out of gas. After a few months, I began to take the other half of the tablet shortly after lunch, which kept me going until quitting time. For the first time in many years, I could work eight or nine hours a day and feel productive for most of them. I will not deny that I was a space case from the moment I yelled, "Honey, I'm home," until I hit the sack, but it was very different from my experience on Adderall, the product of well-deserved mental exhaustion, rather than a result of drug withdrawal.

It was difficult to compare Adderall to Provigil. In terms of reducing my distractibility, I thought they were equally effective. Provigil also seemed to have enhanced my working memory, although I was not the firecracker I had been on Adderall. My visuospatial memory, much improved on Adderall, was as bad as always with Provigil, which did not surprise me: Cognitive domains selectively responsive to dopamine, such as spatial working memory, were unaffected by Provigil, which did not utilize dopaminergic pathways to do its work.

I returned to Jonathan Canick's office to find out how I'd score on the same tests I'd taken before. He was as curious as I was to see what the drug could do for me. The first time he'd asked me to name as many animals as I could in a minute, I'd landed in the thirty-eighth percentile. On Adderall, I was in the eightieth percentile. On Provigil, I had slipped back to the fiftieth percentile. On the test of facial recognition (which I figured I'd nail, since I'd seen these dorky-looking men twice before), the news was the same. Without any drugs, I tested in the nineteenth percentile. With Adderall, I'd made it to the ninety-third. With Provigil, I was in the twenty-seventh percentile, nearly back to the starting point.

Frankly, I was puzzled. Maybe Provigil's impact was subtle. Maybe it didn't manifest itself in these sorts of tests. Still, there were many hours of the day when I experienced unprecedented clarity—a calm alertness that I treasured. I'd play a game I called "race the thesaurus," where I'd ponder for a second over the right word, then click the button on my keypad that took me to Thesaurus.com. If I could come up with the word I wanted before the listings were on the screen, I won. On days when I'd had adequate sleep and Provigil was in my bloodstream, I racked up the big scores. The woman who teaches my exercise class commented that I was much more in synch with the rest of the group. One evening, long after the Provigil had worn off, my book club sat in stunned silence as I rattled off the names of a half dozen characters in Zadie Smith's novel *On Beauty*. Something had obviously changed.

When I got Cephalon's annual report, I saw that unless the world had unexpectedly been flooded with narcoleptics, I wasn't the only one who had noticed the benefit. Between 2002 and 2005, sales of Provigil climbed 51 percent, to $439 million. Compared to Adderall, with sales of $1.16 billion in 2005, it was very small potatoes. But there was no denying it: In the space of six months, Provigil had started to look very interesting. Barbara Sahakian and Danielle Turner, the investigators at Cambridge, told me they expected that it would be remembered not as a drug for the treatment of narcolepsy, but as the forerunner of a new class of pharmaceuticals targeted to the specific molecules that underlie memory and attention. In the spring of 2006, things turned sour for Provigil. Given its excellent results, Cephalon intended to extend the drug's labeling and market it as a treatment for ADHD. But with all the questions that had emerged about Ritalin and Adderall's safety, it was a tough time for attention deficit drugs. When Cephalon's clinical trial hit a snag—one out of 933 children who took part in the trial developed Stevens-Johnson syndrome, a potentially life-threatening skin condition, most likely unrelated to the drug—the FDA turned the pharmaceutical company down. The company has relinquished plans to market Provigil for ADHD in the foreseeable future.

DRUGS IN THE PIPELINE

There are about forty cognition-enhancing drugs in human clinical trials right now, all of them intended to improve wakefulness, attention, memory, decision making and planning. "The idea of cognitive enhancement as a lifestyle choice—I think it's going to change society," said Martha Farah, who directs the Center for Cognitive Neuroscience at the University of Pennsylvania and has written extensively about the topic. "The drugs people currently use to enhance attention—they have non-trivial side effects, but nevertheless, a lot of people are enhancing attention with those drugs. Project that trend ten years into the future, and it's probably going to be very common. I'd definitely like to put my retirement money into that stock." At least a dozen biotechnology companies are feverishly working to produce drugs that may eventually make age-related cognitive impairment a thing of the past. These biotechs, in conjunction with the pharmaceutical companies that are panting to take the most promising compounds off their hands for further development, have their attention fixed on what will be a vast market. According to Harry M. Tracy, who authors the newsletter *Neuroinvestment*, the company that develops a drug to safely improve cognition will rack up sales in the billions. Biotech companies are rushing to identify all the genes involved in memory formation. The goal is to discover drug compounds that can modulate memory by interacting with the protein products of these genes. Most of the drugs fall into one of two categories: They either ramp up neurotransmitters that strengthen memory formation, or they block those that get in the way of the process.

Although there are no inherent regulatory barriers preventing the FDA's approval of medicines that, as one biotech company, Saegis Pharmaceuticals, puts it "protect and enhance the function of the human mind," the agency is unlikely to green-light any drug intended solely for the treatment of midlife memory impairment. The FDA has directed companies pursuing memory drugs to first seek approval for treatment of more serious disorders, such as Alzheimer's disease and mild cognitive impairment, an ill-defined condition that is believed to precede Alzheimer's.

The problem with the FDA's mandate, explains Tracy, is that the agency is mistakenly operating under the assumption that Alzheimer's disease and age-related memory impairment will respond to the same treatments. It may be, he said, that a drug that's effective in stopping age-related memory impairment in its tracks might do nothing at all for Alzheimer's disease, where brain biochemistry is massively disturbed.

Of the compounds currently under development, most work by tweaking the genes that allow nerve cells to move items in working memory to long-term memory, by regulating a complex biochemical pathway that produces changes in the strength and structure of synaptic connections between neurons. This process, which etches permanent connections between nerve cells, is critical for the consolidation of memory. Cortex Pharmaceuticals is developing an ampakine compound that promises to enhance production of BDNF, which as you may recall, acts as a fertilizer for dendritic branches and new cells. In a recent rat study, analysis of hippocampal tissue showed that treated rats had twice as much BDNF in their brain tissue as the control subjects. The elevated levels of BDNF remained for many hours after the drugs had left the animals' bodies. The company, which has already performed several human clinical trials, will begin another one in 2007. Although middle-aged people do experience failures of consolidation, as we have seen, their larger problems lie in deficits of attention and working memory. Many of the drugs currently under development may in fact worsen working memory, according to Amy Arnsten, a neurobiologist at Yale. Certainly, they do nothing to amplify attention and concentration. It's likely, therefore, that more than one drug will be required to address the various aspects of memory loss.

Eric Wasserman, who is head of the brain-stimulation unit at the U.S. National Institute of Neurological Disorders and Stroke, has arrived at a completely different approach to cognitive enhancement. He discovered that passing a small electrical current through the brain, in a process called transcranial direct-current stimulation, boosted verbal and motor skills and improved learning and memory in perfectly healthy people. The overall effect, Wasserman says, is "like giving a cup of coffee to a relatively focal part of the brain." When the current was administered to the left frontal lobe, it boosted by 20 percent subjects' ability to generate a list of words beginning with a given letter.

It's a tiny current, between one and two milliamps, and Wasserman thinks that in due time, you'll be able to buy yourself "a gizmo about the size of an MP3 player" that you can insert into a hat. "Turn it on, and you'll feel better," he said. "Turn it off, and you're back to where you started."

The prospect of cognitive enhancement has thrust ethical concerns into the spotlight. Francis Fukuyama, author of *Our Posthuman Future*, suggests that public policy should restrict research for the purpose of enhancement. "The original purpose of medicine," he wrote, "is to heal the sick, not to turn healthy people into gods." I, for one, am not expecting to develop any godlike abilities. I'd settle for remembering, with perfect clarity, the exact look on my younger son's face when he rushed into the yard to tell me that he had just dropped a half-gallon bottle of maple syrup on the kitchen floor.

The philosophical debate is too ponderous to explore here, but it poses several valid questions. Ought we be able to buy ourselves abilities that eclipse those we were born with? If we're going to live to 120 (and by 2050, quite a few of us will), is it essential that we find a way to supplement our memory and attention? Will the availability of enhancing compounds result in a permanent schism between the cognitive haves and have-nots? Will people feel compelled to take performance-enhancing substances in order to remain competitive in the face of the unrelenting demands of a twenty-four-hour-a-day society? "When a safe and effective method of enhancing memory is available, it's really going to put the squeeze on people," said Martha Farah. "They may have to enhance, or risk being passed over in employment opportunities or competitive school situations." Will there be a time when a commercial pilot, or an air-traffic controller, or a bus driver—someone responsible for the lives of hundreds or thousands of people—will be required to take these drugs or give up his or her job? And most interesting—at least to me: What are the chances that, by taking these drugs, we are monkeying around with a meticulously designed system of forgetting, thereby setting ourselves up to become repositories of useless information, unable to see the forest for the trees?

I wrestled with these enigmas, but my pragmatic self kept butting in, asking who I thought I was kidding. Was there a reason, I wondered, that humans didn't evolve with tons of working memory and total recall? Our big brains already sucked up so much of our fuel in the form of glucose. In millennia past, the demands of an even more capacious brain would have appropriated the energy our ancestors needed for hard physical labor, or even for survival. But for those of us who sat at desks and stared at screens, those days were over. The brain was the winner, hands down. If these drugs were available and considered relatively safe (as safe, say, as Adderall), middle-aged people who planned to live long, active, intellectually demanding lives, who feared the prospect of decades of dependence, would surely find a way to get them into their medicine cabinets.

12

MEDITATION AND NEUROFEEDBACK

· · ·

Going in for a Tune-up: Why Tinkering
with Brain Waves Can Improve Attention

The neurologist who prescribed Provigil had asked me to participate in an eight-week-long program of attentional training called
"mindfulness meditation." He'd feel better, he told me, if he knew that
I was pursuing some fundamental changes in the way I lived.

This method of meditation, I learned, was quite different from the
more familiar mantra approach, where you focused on an object or a
word. In mindfulness, instead of struggling to suppress thoughts, or to
relax, you took notice of thoughts and feelings as they passed through
your consciousness. You did not make judgments about them, elaborate on their implications, or consider whether you needed to take
action. You simply acknowledged the thought, and returned to focus
on your breathing. Because of the emphasis on what was happening
in the here and now, the training taught you how to sustain attention,

and how to shift your focus rapidly from a wayward thought back to the matter at hand—your breath. In time, the theory went, you'd switch out of habitual, automatic patterns of reaction. Instead of getting caught in ruminative, elaborative thought streams—what your boss said, what it might mean, what you should do about it—you'd learn to acknowledge the thought and leave it at that. Once your mind stopped behaving like a runaway horse, you'd have more resources available to deal with your current experience. The bottom line was improved resistance to distraction and augmented working memory.

Mindfulness meditation programs were cropping up all over. Four of my friends, none of them particularly New Age or crunchy, had participated. When they emerged, they reported feeling calmer, happier and more focused. They even slept better. Finding the right instructor was key, they said, or the session could turn into group therapy. Frankly, I wasn't interested in spending eight weeks listening to other people's problems with anxiety and stress. I wanted to deal with my own.

Alan Wallace, president of the Santa Barbara Institute for Consciousness Studies, who often served as a translator for the Dalai Lama during neuroscience conferences, recommended Margaret Cullen, a clinical psychologist who ran the mindfulness-based stress-reduction program at Kaiser Permanente Medical Center in downtown Oakland. For me, it meant a forty-five-minute trip once a week, in rush-hour traffic, and a somewhat shorter trip home in the pitch dark. Wallace assured me that it would be worth it: Cullen was one of the best.

MINDFULNESS IN PRACTICE

For the first session of Intervention #6, I arrived early on an April evening, taking my time as I passed through a lovely courtyard garden filled with lush English roses and bearded irises, all bathed in golden evening light. A patio table and chair, off in one corner, seemed to call to me: Surely, an hour spent here would do me more good than two hours bent up like a pretzel. On the second floor, I found Cullen's classroom. The seven other students were sitting in chairs that formed a semicircle. Several clutched copies of Jon Kabat-Zinn's book, *Full Catastrophe Living*, a text that was assigned for class reading. Cullen, herself middle-aged, impeccably coiffed and manicured, entered the room in understated yoga clothes, her lips forming a gentle smile. It was the end of a long working day and the rest of us were frazzled, but Cullen was calmly alert and very tuned in. I took this as a good sign. I'd dreaded finding myself in the hands of a pathologically laid-back hippie dressed in peasant blouse and Birkenstocks.

She asked each of us—five middle-aged women, two women in their twenties and one thirtyish man—to take turns explaining what we hoped to achieve in the next eight weeks. She discouraged us from going into the specifics of our travails. This was not a therapy group. If anyone needed that kind of help, she'd be happy to talk privately, after class.

I was the only participant who had signed up in the hope of improving my attention and memory. The others were there to deal with stress and pain, both psychological and physical. That was to be expected: When Jon Kabat-Zinn developed the first mindfulness-based stress-reduction program, in 1979 at the University of Massachusetts, his goal was to help patients whose pain symptoms did not respond to conventional medicine.

Mindfulness, Cullen explained, was simply a matter of moment-to-moment awareness. It could be cultivated by purposely paying attention to things that ordinarily wouldn't merit a moment's thought. When you started to pay closer attention, you were likely to see an intrinsic order and connectedness between things that was not apparent before. By paying attention, you literally became more awake.

After a few more introductory remarks, Cullen presented each of us with a single raisin, which we were to eat very slowly, savoring its sweetness and its tartness, observing the way that the wrinkles smoothed out in our mouths. We were not to swallow until she gave the signal. I became quite involved with that raisin. By the time she told us to swallow, I knew it very well.

When it was time to embark on our first meditation, known as a full-body scan, we pulled bolsters, meditation cushions and army blankets from a well-stocked closet. As soon as we lay down on our backs, pillows under our knees, I knew I was in trouble. I had been awake since dawn. I'd taken the second dose of Provigil right after lunch, as was my habit, and it had long since worn off. As soon as Cullen began to guide the meditation, in a tone that was matter-of-fact but still soothing, a soporific wave washed over me. I swam to the surface, only to be hit with another big roller. "Just don't snore," I begged myself, before losing the battle and sinking into unconsciousness.

I woke up to the sound of a sweet little Tibetan chime that resonated for at least thirty seconds.

"How was that?" Cullen asked. I lifted my head and looked around. Everyone seemed deeply fulfilled, rosy, glowing, on his or her way to a new and improved consciousness. Was I the only one, I wondered, who had taken a twenty-minute nap?

I wanted to be able to report to Anthony Chen that this approach was working—that I was becoming focused and attentive, and would not, after all, require a lifelong prescription for Provigil. Each morning, as part of the program, I rose early, inserted my earbuds and prepared to do the requisite half hour of guided meditation and gentle yoga practice. In the subsequent weeks of the class, we expanded our activities, adding chi gung, a fusion of meditation and gentle exercise that I'd seen Chinese octogenarians practice in Huangpu Park in Shanghai. Remembering the order of the movements was tough, but at least I was standing, and remained awake.

It seemed like it should be so easy—inhaling and exhaling. But I was getting an uncomfortably close look at the uproar known as my mind. I recognized that it was hopelessly opportunistic, irrepressibly busy. Back in class, people reported their excellent progress, making me reluctant to talk about my failures. I suspected that I was insufficiently committed. Some had really taken to it, dedicating weekends and extra hours to meditation, even going off on retreats together. They came in bubbling with news of improved concentration and newfound tranquility.

When I finally worked up the nerve to mention my troubles to Margaret Cullen, she told me that it was normal, at certain times, to encounter resistance. Falling asleep, buzzing with thoughts—these qualified, and if I kept at it, they would go away and leave me in peace.

I toyed with the idea of taking Provigil before meditating, but frankly, it seemed redundant. What could possibly be the point of taking a drug that improved attention and focus before pursuing a practice that was supposed to improve attention and focus? Then I read a study noting that, typically, people who have brain injuries that have left them distractible or hyperactive cannot meditate. Neither could people who were chronically sleep deprived; the minute they relaxed, they were out cold. I wished someone had clued me in earlier.

From Alan Wallace, I learned about Susan Smalley's efforts. She was codirector of the Mindful Awareness Research Center (MARC) at UCLA, where she'd developed a meditation program intended for adolescents and adults with ADHD, as an alternative to pharmaceutical treatment. With her colleagues, she'd reframed mindfulness for people whose brains were at least as intractable as mine. The secret, she explained, was to shorten the length of the meditations. There was no way on earth that I was going to be able to sit for a half hour. I should try to sustain my focus for five minutes. When I achieved that, I could move on to ten minutes. It was worth the effort, she told me. Results were still being calculated, but the first group had shown significant improvements on neurocognitive tests that measured attention, as well as a reduction in anxiety and depressive symptoms. The training worked, she said, but I'd have to modify my approach to fit my needs.

I went straight to the MARC Web site, where I found Smalley's quickie meditation practice, which was more my speed. I found something else as well: a description of a pilot study, as yet unfunded, that involved using EEG-based neurofeedback treatment in conjunction with mindfulness training. During a neurofeedback session, electrodes were attached to a patient's scalp, and a monitor displayed neurological activity. All brains produce electrophysiological currents, reflecting the firing speed of neurons. These brain waves, alpha, beta, delta, theta and gamma oscillations, are measurable with electroencephalogram equipment. In a meditative state, high-amplitude gamma waves dominated in the frontal lobes. If those with attention deficits could not achieve meditative brain waves on their own, the pilot study hypothesized, perhaps neurofeedback could nudge them into the right patterns.

I'll admit that it seemed like cheating, but I was sick of finding myself asleep, or even worse, totally absorbed in my shopping list while I was supposed to be meditating. Maybe I could get comfortable in a chair, with some electrodes glued to my scalp, and slip into a meditative state. I could learn to control brain rhythms associated with attention and arousal. Susan Smalley couldn't help me, she admitted. The Mindful Awareness Research Center was interested in neurofeedback, but for now, there was no money for it in the budget.

I got on the Internet and started to look around. Quickly, I realized that few fields are as unregulated as neurofeedback. You need more hours of training to hang out a shingle as a certified massage therapist than you do to glue some electrodes on a person's head and mess around with their brain circuitry. There was a large hooey factor, and it was clear that many psychologists had added neurofeedback to their practices to pump up their incomes. It could be very expensive and time-consuming, requiring an average of forty-one half-hour sessions. Before you could get started, most therapists required a quantitative electroencephalogram (QEEG), which gathered a large amount of data defining how your brain waves differed from the norm.

THE OPTIMIZER

I wasn't very interested in schlepping weekly to a psychologist with a sideline in electrodes. When I found Marvin Sams, an outspoken Texan who specialized in clinical and research EEG, I was intrigued.

Ten years earlier, Sams had developed and patented the Electro-Cap, a Lycra-spandex bathing-cap-style headgear, with the electrodes conveniently sewn into the right places. This new cap immediately replaced the uncomfortable homemade version of elastic bands, hunks of metal and cotton balls. He'd sold the company a few years back and opened the Sams Center for Optimal Performance in Dallas so that he could return to his first love—treating patients.

When we spoke on the phone, I liked his twangy Texas accent, and his inclination to call me "ma'am." In his opinion, neurofeedback did not belong in the hands of psychologists. It was a technical matter, requiring significant expertise in the ways of electroencephalography. Over the last twenty years, there'd been all sorts of progress—easy-to-operate new hardware had come on the market, making it possible for "any Suzy Homemaker to set up shop." But EEG neurofeedback wasn't something you picked up in a long weekend, or, for that matter, in a year's training. "We're dealing with the brain, the most complex system in the known universe," he said, "and we've got people with no expertise out tinkering with it. It's like sending your sixteen-year-old out to fix your Ferrari.

"I want to know how your brain is doing its job," he said. "When I get through talking to your brain, I'll know all about it." His role, as he saw it, was to remediate and optimize brain function. "I'm interested in performance, in efficiency versus inefficiency," he said. Feeling a little bit like I was going in to have my engine overhauled and my shocks replaced, I arranged to fly to Dallas to see him and begin Intervention #7. I'd stay for a week, and have two neurofeedback sessions each day. I'd go home for a week. Then I'd come back, and repeat the process. It would be rigorous, Sams said. At times, I'd feel wiped out, uncomfortably hyperactive, or, his favorite, "tired and wired" at the same time. Most of his patients from out of town stayed at the nearby Bradford Suites, just off the North Dallas Tollway. I'd rise early, work in the morning, trudge off to Sams' office after lunch, and return around half-past four to work some more. We agreed to get started in early January, as soon as a family of four from Australia was all tuned up and ready to head back home. That gave me just enough time to clear Provigil from my system. Marvin Sams insisted on that: He wanted to hear my brain talking to him, loud and clear.

Sams was an appealingly beefy middle-aged man, dressed in a jacket and tie, with a hearty laugh, a courtly manner and a tendency to produce metaphors involving Texas football, which no doubt worked better for his Dallas Cowboys patients than they did for me. His assistant produced the Electro-Cap, and wired me up for a thirteen-channel EEG. He'd look at my brain waves, and then compare them to forty-five years' worth of data, which would show him where my brain deviated from the norm. With that information under his belt, he'd set to correcting the problem.

"Wait," I said. "What if you 'optimize' me and I come out so normal that I can't do my job anymore?"

He'd heard it before, of course. "Believe me," he said, "I'm not about to drain away your creative spark. This will only make it easier for you to put it to work."

The first two tests, IVA and TOVA, Sams described as "the world's hardest video." As he described what I was about to do, it seemed awfully easy: I'd see numbers—ones and twos—flash on the monitor. Simultaneously, I'd hear the numbers spoken. If I heard or saw the number one, I clicked the mouse button. If I heard or saw the number two, I was not to click. There would be 125 auditory cues and 125 visual cues in fifteen minutes, testing thirty-eight variables of impulse control and attention. Right away, I noticed that I seemed to have little control over my responses. My mouse finger had a mind of its own. I began to moan. At the end, Sams flicked on the lights and patted me sympathetically on the shoulder. While we waited, the printer spat out my results: a working diagnosis of attention-deficit hyperactivity disorder, brought on, at least in part, by a significant brain trauma to the right frontal region.

"How on earth can it tell?" I asked him.

"It's all right here," he said. He waved two densely printed pages at me. I glanced at the two-point type and the parade of unfamiliar words—"absolute amplitude," "relative power," "compressed spectral array"—and decided I'd leave the interpretation to him.

Although my visual attention was only moderately hindered, my auditory attention was severely impaired. There was nothing wrong with my hearing per se, Sams explained; no doubt I'd pass a hearing test just fine. It was a matter of processing, achingly difficult to tease out without a test like IVA. From what he saw, he imagined I took a very long time to process verbal instructions. I probably had no idea, much of the time, what people were saying to me. In addition, my unwieldy mouse finger reflected my brain's inability to control my impulses. I knew I wasn't supposed to click on those twos, but I did it anyway.

After some further testing, Sams gave me the news at a small round table in the corner of the training room. My brain, he indicated, was slumped in an alpha state. I had alpha waves all over the place, in regions where I'd be better off with theta and beta. He wasn't surprised—people with ADHD and brain injuries tended to have excessive alpha in the frontal lobes, creating problems with concentration and memory. With so much alpha, my brain was stuck in neutral, relaxed and disengaged, neither working nor sleeping. I also had too much posterior and frontal delta, at the frequency normally experienced during sleep, and some theta, which was associated with mental inefficiency.

He'd place a bet that I was usually locked in a drowsy state—that it took a whole lot to rev up my engine. He'd venture a guess that I'd developed some techniques for overcoming this woozy condition. I probably needed to work myself up into an anxious frenzy in order to get out of the gate. The look on my face must have told him he'd nailed it.

"What about gamma?" I said brightly. "Gamma's what you want in order to get into a meditative state."

"Do you plan to sit in a cave for the next thirty years?" he asked. "Because that's the only reason for you to be in a meditative state. Gamma's not about optimizing performance. It's not about being prepared to rock 'n' roll. I doubt that gamma is what you need. If you get neurofeedback in the right way, you're not going to need meditation."

I'd come all the way to Dallas to improve my meditation skills, I told him. Sams told me not to worry. My brain was about to go to his gym. He'd tone it up. He'd teach it to engage, instead of slacking off in alpha rhythms. I'd feel brighter and more bushy-tailed with more beta, which would allow me to focus and stay on task. He'd do this, he explained, by plying my neurons with various audio tones while I played the game of Tetris on a Game Boy so ancient it was held together with masking tape. If he'd told me that he intended to treat me by speaking in tongues and dancing naked around a campfire, I couldn't have been more skeptical.

Sams explained that playing Tetris was in fact an extremely complex task. It involved memory, strategy, planning and concentration, as well as the all-important capacity to be able to flip the puzzle pieces upside down and around in your mind, all while constantly moving your thumbs.

Over the ten days of my treatment, I played so much Tetris that I saw geometric shapes falling into place before my eyes not only when I was sleeping, but while I was driving. An experienced Tetris player racks up at least twenty-five thousand points in a game, but when I started, I was amazingly bad, even for me. My scores hovered around ninety. While I played, Sams monitored my EEG on his computer monitor. I was concentrating so hard on what was going on under my thumbs that I was hardly aware of what he was doing. I'd score poorly for game after game, and then suddenly, I'd rack up the triple digits. Minutes later, I'd be struggling to make it to sixty points before the game ended. I noticed that Sams kept his eye on my little Nintendo screen, but it took days for me to catch on: As he manipulated frequencies, he was giving my brain information, telling it how it could perform better. He could improve or diminish my performance, as he wished.

Late each afternoon, I left Sams' office and crawled back to the Bradford Suites, so blitzed that getting any work done was out of the question. The best I could do was to put my dinner in the microwave and watch really dumb shows on television. My nights were even more sleepless than usual. "That happens," Sams said, when I told him. "When we finally get the brain out of neutral and into drive, it tends to zoom off uncontrollably for a little while."

Ten days after I'd started, Marvin Sams put me through the same tests he'd administered at the beginning of our time together. This time, I decided to go for accuracy rather than speed. During the IVA and the TOVA, I tried to get a grip on my mouse finger. I clicked only when I was absolutely sure that I was seeing and hearing the number one. When the results spewed from the printer, my scores on the two tests had gone way up, into the normal range in all areas except the test of auditory attention. Even there, I'd improved: Now I was only moderately impaired. The results no longer supported a diagnosis of ADHD, Sams said, but I was to proceed with caution. After two weeks of intensive training, my brain was in a state of chaos. We wouldn't know for sure where I stood until I'd given it a couple of weeks to reset. And I'd show significantly more improvement if I had six to ten more sessions. Effectively, I was leaving in a half-baked state.

There was a car outside, waiting to take me to the airport, I said. The additional sessions would have to wait. That was no problem, Sams said. The next time I came through Texas, we could finish up. I promised to think about a visit to Austin in bluebonnet season.

Back in California, I observed my own behavior, to see if anything had changed. After a total of ten days on the road, I'd returned to a really sticky kitchen floor and children who had outgrown all their pants. How was I handling it? Was I more focused when I was making pancakes? Were there more words at my disposal? I thought I sensed a neural perkiness that I'd previously associated with pharmaceutical-grade stimulants. Perhaps it was only evidence of the placebo effect, but I embraced it. I took the Provigil out of my purse and put it away in the medicine cabinet. Maybe I'd need it again, but for now, I was okay.

A couple of days after I returned, I snatched up my earbuds and sat down to listen to the short meditation that Susan Smalley had put on the MARC Web site. I listened carefully to the instructions. Inhale. Exhale. Inhale. Exhale. I avoided thinking about whether or not I was producing sufficient gamma waves. Five minutes went by quickly. I never thought of the shopping list. Ten minutes passed, without any intercranial discussion of the day's schedule. At eleven minutes, I was still awake, but so were the kids and the dogs and it was time to make breakfast. Every little bit helped, I told Sams when he called to check up on me. I'd be back in Texas as soon as my schedule allowed. The time had come to tackle the big one—sleep.

13

I'LL SLEEP WHEN I'M DEAD

· · ·

Sacrifice Your Slumber and You'll Perform
as Well as if You've Had a Few Stiff Drinks

I yearn for sleep. I treasure it. I just can't get it," admitted Kevin, who used to slumber for nine hours at a clip. "I've become a much worse sleeper as I age. A typical night is two hours awake, from three to five. Thank God for *CNN Headline News*."

Like Kevin, you've probably noticed that you sleep fewer hours, and not nearly as well as you did a couple of decades ago. On average, the time spent conked out declines by twenty-seven minutes each decade—so if you averaged seven hours in your early twenties, you're likely to be down to five and a half hours a night by the time you turn fifty. About forty-two million sleeping pill prescriptions were filled in 2006, up nearly 60 percent since 2000, building a market that is currently worth $2.1 billion each year. In that period, prescriptions for sleeping pills written for people between the ages of 44 and 65 increased by 62 percent. These numbers surely suggest that a lot of people don't get enough shut-eye.

Recent studies suggest hours of sleep decline in midlife because you become more sensitive to the sleep-disturbing effects of stress hormones. A kick of adrenaline (the midnight phone call) resulting in a slightly elevated level of cortisol that wouldn't have bothered you back in college will keep you wide awake in middle age. As other hormones that keep the metabolism on an even keel (including estrogen and testosterone) begin to decline, cortisol gains the upper hand.

Conventional wisdom dictates that you need less sleep as you age. It isn't true: Unless you get eight hours, or very close to it, your brain feels the pinch. Sleep deprivation affects sustained attention, spatial learning, processing speed and accuracy, working memory and reaction time—in short, it hammers every one of your cognitive abilities.

"One complete night of sleep deprivation is as impairing in simulated driving tests as a legally intoxicating level of blood alcohol," reported Mark Mahowald, a professor of neurology at the University of Minnesota. Nor do you need to stay up all night to act as if you've tied one on: Have yourself two or three late nights and early mornings (maybe right before your deadline for a big presentation) and you'll be as savvy as a guy with three Scotch and sodas under his belt. "When I am tired," explained George, a high school math teacher, "I find that I don't have sufficient wits to keep the subject matter and the level of the kids' understanding in mind at the same time. I either forget what I'm doing or what they're capable of learning. I have realized that it is often better for me to get to class with enough sleep rather than staying up half the night to score the tests."

The average adult now sleeps 6.9 hours on weeknights and an hour more on weekends, about 20 percent less than he slept in 1900. There are loads more reasons to stay up. There's the siren song of the Internet, of course, but gyms are also open around the clock, as are 1,300 Wal-Marts, 237 Home Depots, and nearly all FedEx Kinkos facilities. At the Apple store in Manhattan, you can get your computer fixed or buy a new iPod twenty-four hours a day. The lure dangles before us—if we just ignore our circadian rhythms, we'll get more done and have time for fun. In a study conducted by the National Sleep Foundation, two-thirds of the subjects reported that sleepiness interfered with their concentration, and estimated that the quality of their work, when sleepy, declined by 30 percent.

Daytime sleepiness is so common that people take it for granted. They shouldn't, observed David Dinges, who heads the sleep and chronobiology division at the University of Pennsylvania. "What people are experiencing," he said, "are bouts of microsleep, and these are far from normal." Each time you have to remind yourself to snap to attention, to quit operating on autopilot, you're under the spell of a brain that has succumbed to the irrepressible homeostatic urge to sleep. "People have all sorts of ways of explaining it to themselves," Dinges observed. "They tell themselves that they're falling asleep because they've had a heavy meal, because the lights are low, because it's too warm in the room, or because they're bored. They're wrong, all around. They're falling asleep because they are carrying a sleep debt that their bodies are determined to fix."

Although catching a quick nap isn't the same as descending into several solid sleep cycles, there's no question that it will help sharpen you up fast. In multiple studies, investigators have demonstrated that napping after learning something new significantly increases your mastery. In a study at the Salk Institute for Biological Studies, nappers mastered a computer game 50 percent faster than those who stayed awake. The Japanese are so convinced of the benefits of napping that the country's Ministry of Health, Labor and Welfare recently recommended that people nap twenty to thirty minutes before 3:00 P.M. to boost health and work efficiency. Indeed, napping may be a hallmark of efficiency: The Germans are the world's most prolific nappers—one out of five naps three times a week. A nap of under thirty minutes is most restorative. Any longer than an hour, and you may start to behave like a siesta-taking Spaniard, inclined to stay up until 3:00 A.M.

Whether sleep deprivation is volitional, emerging from your desire to add hours to your day, or stems from chronic insomnia, the body perceives more than a day or two of a sleep shortage as an all-fired emergency. Accordingly, it activates the hotline to the HPA axis, triggering the stress response, which calls for the red-alert approach to blood-glucose regulation, flooding the heart and the muscles, while ignoring the brain. Stressed-out hippocampal neurons go into survival mode. They stop producing brain-derived neurotropic factor (BDNF), resulting in a sharp decrease in neurogenesis. The sleep-deprived body becomes insensitive to insulin, increasing the risk of hypertension, obesity, diabetes and memory loss.

INSOMNIA IS COMMON IN MIDLIFE

That was alarming news for me and my sleepless comrades. So many of us were "up all night" that we'd discussed the feasibility of designing a special kind of switchboard intended for the bedside table, one that would light up to show you which of your friends were wide awake and ready for a chat. According to a National Sleep Foundation poll, 63 percent of American women and 54 percent of men say that they experience symptoms of insomnia at least a few days a week, while chronic insomnia affects about 15 percent of the population. "Why can't the brain just go off to dreamland, like it used to?" wondered Melissa, the freelancer, who started waking up at 4:00 A.M. in her early forties. "Why does it have to feel responsible?"

"Clearly, there's a special little corner of the brain dedicated to niggling anxieties," observed Robert Stickgold, who studies sleep at Harvard Medical School. "What does the brain think it is accomplishing as it runs the same fruitless loop over and over? There's never any progress, and when you finally drag yourself out of bed in the morning, you've lost hours of shut-eye to circular thinking." He concludes that this relentless situation exists because you're in a semisleep state where the prefrontal cortex is inactivated, leaving such useful capacities as logic and decision making off-line.

To get deep into REM sleep, you must pass through four stages of what scientists imaginatively call "non-REM." If your sleep architecture is normal, you run through the process—non-REM, followed by REM, four to six times per night, at 90 to 120 minutes a pop.

If you're interrupted at any point—say, your wife kicks you in the shins and you wake up, or your elevated cortisol level jerks you out of slumber—you have to start over. Perform a quick calculation—say, five cycles a night at 100 minutes each—that's 500 minutes. Divide by sixty, if you still can, and you'll see why close to eight hours are necessary.

Stages three and four of non-REM are called "slow-wave sleep." Slow-wave sleep gives the brain the chance to extract meaning from the tons of jumbled information that comes at it during the day. It helps the hippocampus establish memories of events—the details and flow of your meeting with your boss—and set them in context. Slow-wave is equally important in solidifying procedural memories—how, exactly, you log into that database, and what it is that you're supposed to do once you get there. Because the brain is able to run through all the events that have occurred during the day and look for interesting juxtapositions, slow-wave sleep enhances creativity.

Thus, it is very bad news that slow-wave sleep, which constitutes nearly 20 percent of your slumber in early adulthood, diminishes to just over 3 percent of your sleep in middle age. By age forty-five, according to the authors of a University of Chicago study, most men have completely lost the ability to generate slow-wave sleep. Researchers suspect that the falloff in cognitive abilities that we perceive in our midforties is primarily due to this reduction. Levels of thyroid hormone and growth hormone, both secreted during slow-wave sleep, drop off right along with it.

No one knows why slow-wave sleep disappears, but one thing's for sure: Everyone wants it back. Several pharmaceutical companies are currently tweaking drugs that promise to restore slow-wave sleep. These next-generation sleeping pills won't put you to sleep faster, or make you sleep longer—they'll simply improve the quality of your downtime by increasing your slow-wave sleep by about 20 percent. Theoretically, you could exist on fewer hours of much higher quality sleep, a prospect that holds some attraction for the chronically busy.

REM sleep occurs when cortisol is lowest. If your cortisol remains elevated all night instead of peaking in early morning hours as part of the body's physiological response to awakening, you may not be getting much REM sleep. You'll wake unrefreshed and not a lot smarter than you were when you went to bed. REM is the cleanup crew, brought in to sweep up the detritus that remains after slow wave finishes its gig. In REM, the brain examines the just processed material, deciding what to keep and what to toss. If there's been little or no slow-wave sleep, the cleaners can make some terrible mistakes, carting tomorrow's carefully prepared speech off in a Dumpster. REM sleep fosters pattern recognition; when you're low on REM, your mental mapping skills go awry and you lose your way, both literally and figuratively. Decision making also benefits from REM, probably because it allows the brain to integrate information it absorbed during the day but didn't get around to processing until things quieted down late at night.

In Gabriel García-Márquez's novel *One Hundred Years of Solitude*, a plague of insomnia strikes the Colombian village of Macondo. Gradually, it causes people to forget everything—including the names and uses of the most common objects. The sleepless villagers are reduced to labeling everything with an inked brush. They even hang a sign on the cow: "This is the cow. She must be milked every morning so that she will produce milk, and the milk must be boiled in order to be mixed with coffee to make coffee and milk."

Many days, I felt like I ought to get out a Sharpie and start writing my own labels before it was too late. My insomnia, it seemed, operated as a classically conditioned response. I reacted to the slightest noise or environmental alteration by waking up. If the blind flapped against the window shade, I was up. If my neighbors came home from a late party and ran their car's headlights through my bedroom window, I was awake. And usually, I couldn't get back to sleep. It was hard to believe that I was the same person who for years had slept like a rock on the fifteenth floor of an apartment building on West Seventy-second Street in Manhattan, where fire engines tore past all night long, sirens blaring.

Several nights a week, I lay awake from three until five in the morning, waiting for the alarm clock to go off. Sometimes I got up and read, or—figuring there was no point in wasting time—I turned on the computer and went to work. I'd developed a distrustful relationship with sleep. I never knew when, or even if, it would show up. If I didn't sleep, I couldn't work, and I had to work.

Dharma Singh Khalsa's regimen of vitamins and supplements eradicated my insomnia—but only for a couple of months. That was long enough to remind me of how I had felt, in the years before children, when eight hours were typical and I slept in on the weekends. With sufficient sleep, the fog abated and I felt far more focused. I recalled the nearly forgotten pleasure of choosing from a range of appropriate words rather than scratching for meager pickings. I could remember what I intended to do for long enough to actually accomplish it.

And then, as quickly as it had departed, the insomnia was back. Because I knew what was possible, it was worse than before. Sleep was like a lover who teased me, coming and going, bestowing gifts that were sometimes mine—and sometimes not. I could feel the difference; once again, life rubbed me raw. I had to "get the sleep thing handled," as so many doctors had already told me.

It wasn't as if I hadn't tried.

I'd gone the route of relaxing baths and warm milk. I'd done restorative yoga—which I found too stimulating—and meditation that, since I generally fell asleep, had much the same effect as a nice nap. I'd tried melatonin, valerian and L-trytophan, none of which were effective for more than a few days. Neither Ambien nor Sonata worked. They're indicated for seven to ten days, tops, but for me, they worked for only three to five hours during the night before they puttered out. And at three days, they quit working entirely, leaving me awake and anxious, experiencing a highly undesirable treatment-related adverse effect of sleeping pills known as rebound insomnia. A person who has a little trouble getting to sleep once or twice a month is an ideal candidate for sleeping pills. But chronic insomnia is very different: If pills were going to work, you'd need to take them every night. Even if the hypnotic sedatives had done the trick, drugs were not a long-term solution for me.

SLEEPING AT STANFORD

I'd made an appointment to see Tracy Kuo, a psychologist at the Stanford University Sleep Disorder Center, who specializes in behavioral sleep medicine. Sleep medicine, which scientists at Stanford pioneered, is over three decades old, but Kuo's discipline—sleep psychology—is embryonic. (Given the statistics on sleeplessness, it's no surprise that private sleep-medicine clinics are burgeoning. The majority of these clinics are run by neurologists and pulmonary specialists who address sleep-related troubles like obstructive sleep apnea, restless leg syndrome and periodic movement disorder. At least until recently, doctors at these clinics held that insomnia did not exist as an independent condition, but instead emerged from depression, pain or some other disorder.)

In 2000, Kuo came to Stanford as a postdoc. She was fresh out of Richard Bootzin's lab at the University of Arizona. Bootzin, a professor of psychology and psychiatry at the Arizona Sleep Center, and his colleagues took a different view of chronic insomnia. They saw it as a twenty-four-hour physiological problem with a strong psychological component. Instead of growing sleepy at bedtime, Bootzin observed, insomniacs became agitated. Their adrenaline and cortisol levels shot up. Their hearts beat faster. He called it "conditioned hyperarousal." Sending them to bed at a "decent" hour to get a good night's sleep was not the solution. More hours in bed were the last thing an insomniac needed. Bootzin and his investigators (among them, Tracy Kuo) hypothesized that the answer resided instead in sleep restriction—drastically limiting the time a person spent in bed, until the body's homeostatic demand for sleep took over and normal circadian rhythms emerged, maybe for the first time in years. In Bootzin's lab, the principles of cognitive behavioral therapy for insomnia—CBT-I— evolved. Kuo packed them up and took them to Stanford, where she's continued to hone them for half a decade.

Cognitive behavioral therapy is used to treat a variety of problems, including obsessive-compulsive disorders and many types of phobias. The idea behind CBT is quite simple: Alter the behavior that causes the disorder (no more hand washing or flicking of light switches) and the disorder will go away.

CBT-I is so rigorous that a patient must be highly motivated. One study of CBT-I programs showed that 30 percent of patients dropped out in the first few weeks. It's easy to see why. In the beginning, the time you're permitted to sleep is often reduced to the bare minimum—around two hundred minutes, or just over three hours. When you sleep 90 percent of that time, you are allowed to add time, in fifteen-minute increments. In theory, it's possible to do CBT-I on your own. You could set up a schedule and stick with it. But I knew that I wouldn't be able to pull it off without one hell of a cheerleader on my side.

Within a few minutes of meeting Tracy Kuo at Stanford, I knew I had one. Her patients, several of whom had taken the time to speak to me, referred to her as "the goddess of sleep," which led me to expect someone tall, stately and dressed (appropriately enough) in a bedsheet. Instead, I found a bright, poised, expressive young woman with a great big smile, whom I could easily imagine with a brightly colored pompom in each hand. In Kuo, I'd found my cheering squad, and I was ready for Intervention #8.

A few days before my appointment with Kuo, I interviewed one of her CBT-I patients, fifty-four-year-old Maureen. Kuo warned me that when I was through with Maureen, I'd feel as though I'd just sat through an infomercial for CBT-I. It didn't always go so well, Kuo cautioned. It was hard work, and Maureen was extremely motivated. But she thought I should see what success looked like.

Two years earlier, Maureen's fifty-year-old husband died of liver cancer. He passed away only a few brief months after his diagnosis. Her mother and her father died shortly thereafter, leaving her with intractable insomnia. "I just forgot how to sleep," she said. "But I had a teenage son to raise, and I drove around all day for my job as a pharmaceutical sales rep. I was really afraid I'd have an accident. I couldn't afford to let anything happen to me. I had to be at the top of my game."

She'd had several near misses by the time she sat down with Tracy

Kuo. "It was just unbelievable what I would do. I forgot about reports my boss wanted. I lost files he gave me. One day, I parked the car and went into the supermarket, only to find that I had a lady chasing me to tell me that I'd left the car door wide open, with my purse sitting on the seat."

For three months, Maureen saw Tracy Kuo privately, once a week. She'd been getting into bed at nine, staring at the ceiling all night, and getting out at seven, but Kuo cut her back to three hundred minutes—five hours in bed.

The first thing she had to learn, Kuo told Maureen, was how to protect her sleep. "It's harder than you'd expect," Maureen said, "especially when you have a teenager who likes to come into your room at 11:45 and tell you that he's gotten an F on his math test. It takes a lot to say, 'Good night, I'm not going to talk to you about this now,' especially since it is a known fact that teenagers only want to talk to you at midnight."

For Maureen, CBT-I worked. Within a few months, she was sleeping straight through, seven hours a night. Her cognitive symptoms disappeared. "Talk about the fountain of youth," she said. "I felt so great, so much livelier and smarter. My sleep is so delicious now. I'd gotten to the point where I dreaded going to bed, and hated the prospect of waking up in the middle of the night and thinking about all that stuff. Now I look forward to going to sleep. It's better than chocolate cake." She had so much energy that she was going to the gym, taking voice lessons and playing the piano. She'd had to retrain on two of her company's products, which involved taking part in a seven-hour seminar packed with technical information. "I scored 98 percent on the test," Maureen told me. "I know that if I hadn't done CBT-I, I would have remained stressed all day and all night. I think it would have killed me."

Kuo was right: I did feel as if I'd sat through a very persuasive infomercial.

"It's important to impart hope," Kuo said, as we walked down the hall to her office. "Any patient who comes to me has been to many doctors over the years. They're disillusioned, and very tired. I want them to know that fixing this is possible."

Most of Kuo's patients—nearly all of whom are between the ages of forty-five and fifty—match a profile that she calls the "Silicon Valley Classic." The person leads a profoundly irregular life, with fluctuating bedtimes and wake-up times. For them, "There's no structure and no schedule," Kuo explained, "except that which is demanded by work, family and social life. These people are always dealing with time as a limited resource. They see sleep as time they can borrow against, with the expectation that they will catch up eventually. In effect, they train themselves not to be able to sleep."

When patients come to see Kuo, they've typically suffered from insomnia for ten years. Like me, long ago they exhausted the herbal remedies. Most have done time on the harder stuff—swallowing benzodiazepines like Xanax and Ativan, as well as various antide-pressants, non-benzo hypnotics like Ambien and Sonata, and antipsy-chotic drugs such as Zyprexa and Neurontin. "If you go to an M.D.," she said, "and complain of insomnia, you'll come away with a pre-scription. It's what they know. Patients come to me when none of it's working any longer, or they can't stand the cognitive fuzziness asso-ciated with these pharmaceuticals. Often they arrive so loaded with medicine that it takes time to get off."

Most people are capable of establishing a natural rhythm of sleep-ing and wakefulness, she explained. "The first thing you're going to need to do," Kuo said, once we were comfortable in her office, "is to learn to land your helicopters." Once the meaning of her metaphor dawned in my tired brain, I saw what she intended. When I got in bed, I used the downtime as an opportunity to consider various disturbing possibilities. High over my head, the whirlybirds circled, making a tremendous ruckus. "You can't go to sleep if you have those helicop-ters hovering," she explained. "You have to set them down."

Sleep, she explained, was an automatic state. The moment you find yourself having to attend to it, you're in trouble. You're bringing con-sciousness to unconsciousness and those two states are fundamentally incompatible. In order to go off to sleep and stay there for the appropriate number of hours, you have to relinquish control, vigilance and the feelings of dread and frustration you experience when you've had a long string of bad nights. "All of those represent the phenomenon of arousal," Kuo said, "and are incompatible with sleep. Even 'trying' to sleep is self-defeating. You can't just say to a person, 'Quit thinking.' But the problem-solving mind is not the sleeping mind."

My sleep, which Kuo described as very inefficient and short, was no longer my responsibility. She was taking it out of my hands. She assigned what was for me a wildly late bedtime—11:30 P.M.—and told me to set my alarm clock for exactly six hours later. I'd chart my progress in a sleep diary, keeping track of hours awake and hours asleep. As soon as I could sleep for six hours straight, I'd go to bed fifteen minutes earlier. Eventually, Kuo said, I'd sleep for eight hours.

The real challenge, she explained, was what came before bedtime. My job was to start to tell my body when it was time to simmer down. At 10:15, I'd begin to "ramp down," setting the dimmer switch as low as it could go, while still permitting me to read. Even the most brief exposure to bright lights—a quick trip to the bathroom, for instance—would reset my very sensitive body clock, inadvertently alerting it that day had dawned.

"You have to learn to protect your sleep," Kuo said. "You will find that no one else in your house thinks this is a good idea."

She was right, of course. The first night that I threw everyone out of the bedroom (including my husband, whose laptop screen was glowing brightly), I thought I'd spark a revolution. My older son could not believe that I would not help him study for his Spanish final. My younger son, who arrived home late from Little League and had been engaged in homework ever since, woefully pointed out that he hadn't seen me all day. Kuo was right: Protecting my sleep was going to be tough.

And yet there was something really lovely about that quiet time. In truth, I relished it. I could read *Real Simple* and discover all the newest ways to organize the bathroom without feeling guilty that it wasn't my normal bedtime reading, the always stimulating *New York*

Times, which Kuo had put on the forbidden list. The real challenge came after I'd been reading for about ten minutes. My eyelids slid lower and lower. That was a problem, because I wasn't allowed to get into bed and go to sleep for nearly an hour. For a couple of weeks, it was torture. I got up and walked around in my darkened room. When 11:15 finally arrived, and I was allowed to climb into bed, I was asleep in seconds.

Within a few weeks, I was dependably getting five and a half hours, so little that it left me blitzed. I was falling asleep in front of the computer at nine in the morning. With Kuo's blessing, I pulled the Provigil out of the bathroom cabinet to combat what was undeniably a case of excessive daytime sleepiness. It was time, Kuo told me, to start to edge closer to six. I managed that, but when I set the clock for six and a half hours, I stalled. Once again, I began waking up in the middle of the night. My job, when that happened, was to get up and read something even less stimulating than *Real Simple* until I felt sleepy again. Some nights, I was up for a couple of hours.

When Kuo looked over my sleep diary at my third visit, I could tell from her face that something was wrong. "You need more sleep," she said. "You're not going to resolve your cognitive problems on only six hours. And if you start waking up in the middle of the night, you're going to be back to square one."

She suspected that there was something else going on—something that disturbed my sleep if I slipped even slightly over six hours. I didn't fit the profile for obstructive sleep apnea, which affects 4 percent of middle-aged men and 2 percent of middle-aged women, all of whom snore loudly, go silent for a period of up to ten seconds (when they stop breathing), gasp and return to snoring. Nearly all obstructive sleep apnea patients are overweight, or at least heavily jowled, with a large neck circumference. I was slender, and my jaw remained as chiseled as any on Mount Rushmore. There were no reports of snoring from my side of the bed.

Upper airway resistance syndrome could nevertheless exist in non-snoring women like me, with a low body mass and thin, elongated necks, Kuo said. A Finnish study noted that such troubles existed in

17 percent of women, most of whom shared certain physical charac-teristics: a very slim neck, matched with a very high arched palate and a small triangular chin. Many of these women were diagnosed with chronic fatigue syndrome when in fact the struggle for air was waking them up. The key symptoms were identical to those of obstructive sleep apnea: excessive daytime sleepiness, lack of energy, low initia-tive, difficulties in concentration and poor memory, brought on by a combination of oxygen deprivation and virtually no REM sleep.

She wanted me to have a diagnostic sleep study in the Stanford Sleep Disorder Center, she told me. I'd come in around 7:00 P.M. and they'd glue electrodes on my scalp and body. They'd slip wires up my shirtsleeves and down my pants legs and put me to bed. While I snoozed, they'd test every aspect of my sleep physiology. If there were breathing troubles, even subtle ones, the technicians would be able to pinpoint them on the polysomnographic monitoring equipment. The experts at Stanford would take a long look at my sleep architecture. If I did have airway trouble, there were ways to treat it.

A sleep study was the next step, she said. It was up to me to decide if I wanted to take it. If I did not, she warned, I would suffer—indeed, had already suffered—from continued stress created by sleep depri-vation. Not for a moment should I fool myself into thinking that six hours of sleep was enough for any human being. I didn't have the "sleep thing" handled yet, but with the progress I'd made, I knew it was critical to continue to pursue it. This one was just going to take a little more time. In the meanwhile, I'd lined up some other suspects likely to be responsible for causing cognitive impairment.

14

RECREATIONAL DRUGS, ALCOHOL AND OTHER NEUROTOXINS

. . .

The Cognitive Consequences of What You Smoke,

Drink, Eat and Breathe

Mark, now a high school chemistry teacher with two grown children, smoked marijuana for the better part of the 1970s. "All day, every day," he said. "I was out of it for most of a decade." He still smoked a couple of joints a week, "just socially, the way that someone else might have a few drinks." In the last several years, he'd started to have memory problems. It took at least the first three months of every school year for him to get a handle on his student roster. If his lesson plan wasn't in front of him, he blanked on the topics he was required to cover in a unit of instruction. Sometimes, when he forgot how to do a very complex problem, his honor students had to help him out. He'd thought of marijuana as benign, especially when compared to the booze he believed had hastened his father's early descent into Alzheimer's disease. He never touched alcohol, but he was starting to wonder. Could the large amount of pot he'd smoked in his youth—or the pot he occasionally smoked now—be the explanation for the blips in his memory?

It was possible, I told him. A study recently published in *Neurology* showed that long-term marijuana users, who smoked four or more joints a week for ten years, performed significantly below the norm on tests where they were asked to remember a series of words. Even moderate marijuana use could impair working memory by as much as 20 percent. Response time slows, as does the ability to remember the details of events. Heavy marijuana users experienced reduced blood flow in the hippocampus and displayed abnormalities in the small blood vessels of the brain, equal to those that exist in individuals with chronic high blood pressure and diabetes.

Once again, the ever vulnerable hippocampus suffered. A healthy hippocampus is studded with acetylcholine receptors, ready to receive these neurotransmitters, so crucial for learning and memory. THC, the active ingredient in marijuana, confuses the hippocampus, leading it to embrace cannabinoid molecules instead. With insufficient acetylcholine, information stopped short, failing to make it from the frontal lobes into the hippocampal circuit.

Mark was lucky he came of age in the early seventies, I told him: Any later and he might have been a club kid, popping Ecstasy, which was considerably more dangerous. In 1976, Alexander Shulgin, a psychopharmacological researcher, retrieved MDMA, a synthetic union of psychedelics and amphetamines, from obscurity. By 1985, it was so popular among students that the U.S. Drug Enforcement Agency placed an immediate ban on the drug, instantly making it the drug of choice. By dramatically increasing production of serotonin, Ecstasy generates a euphoric high, lasting six to twenty-four hours. In frequent users, it can cause irreversible damage to the central nervous system, resulting in the death of nerve cells. It forces open the blood-brain barrier, allowing larger molecules that don't belong there to enter the brain. The hippocampus and frontal lobes appear to be most vulnerable to the drug's neurotoxic effects, provoking deficits in executive function. In 2003, a team at the University of Newcastle in the UK found that those who had used Ecstasy at least ten times were 23 percent more likely to experience memory problems than those who were drug free. The brain that had seen too much Ecstasy, the study reported, looked much older than it was. Significant areas of tissue had been destroyed.

THE EFFECTS OF ALCOHOL

When used in extreme moderation—maximum health benefits are derived from one half to one serving a day—alcohol can increase the odds that you'll make it to old age without developing Alzheimer's disease. In small amounts, alcohol can lower your risk for heart attack, diabetes, osteoporosis and other forms of mental decline. The truth is that few regular drinkers indulge so sparingly and predictably: They're more likely to knock back a couple of beers or a half bottle of wine with dinner, a few times a week.

That can be a problem: Beginning with just one or two drinks, alcohol produces detectable memory impairments. "It is abundantly clear to me," observes John, the cardiologist who forgot to attend his aunt's funeral, "that splitting a half bottle of wine between two people at dinner every night results in both working and long-term memory loss."

Aaron White, a thirtyish assistant professor of research at Duke University, studies alcoholic blackouts, which are much more common among social drinkers than people assume. ("Blacking out" means that, although you are three sheets to the wind, you are perfectly conscious and unfortunately able to engage in a wide variety of goal-directed, voluntary and often complicated behaviors, including driving cars and having sex. Blacking out should not be confused with "passing out," which involves a loss of consciousness, and could be a great deal safer.) As part of his research, White recorded signals in rats from the CA-1 pyramidal cells, which stand at the gates of the hippocampus. "What I found is that alcohol basically shuts these cells off," he explained when I visited him at Duke. "Drink, and it's the equivalent of not having a hippocampus. You can keep stuff going short-term. You can access old stuff, so you're perfectly capable of dredging up some old grudge and starting an argument. But you can't get a grip on current activities, because the hippocampus is a dead end; it's out of the game. The fundamental defect is the inability to transfer new information from short- to long-term storage."

In mice, continuous consumption of alcohol for as little as eight weeks produced cognitive deficits that lasted for up to twelve weeks after the drinking stopped. If a parallel can be drawn to humans, it suggests that a person who drinks six to eight bottles of beer or one bottle of wine a day for six years can expect to experience learning and memory deficits for up to nine years after he or she stops drinking.

There is no need to be drunk, or even tipsy, to find your memory sidelined; a single heavy dose of alcohol—the stiff G and T you knocked back while you were still searching for the hors d'oeuvres—would do it. Working memory deficits are common, as is a decrease in executive function. "At .15 percent blood concentration of alcohol," White noted, "impairment is small, but it's definitely there, creating what we call 'cocktail party deficits.'" Evelyn, a singer-songwriter, found out the hard way at a New Year's Eve party she gave with her husband. "I had a few glasses of champagne over the course of five or so hours," she said. "Several days later, I had a meeting with a friend who had joined us that night. She brought up a topic that we had apparently covered in some detail at the party. I didn't remember discussing the subject at all, and instantly felt very foolish and vulnerable."

"I think it's pretty self-evident that alcohol dims the memory and intellectual abilities," noted Kevin, the screenwriter. "My daughter loves it when I have a glass of wine while we play each other in chess." With age, alcohol's effect on GABA neural receptors becomes more pronounced, slowing communications between neurons, often to a point where a middle-aged person must struggle to remain awake after only a couple of drinks. Some rats have a gene mutation that makes them exceptionally sensitive to alcohol, leading to rapid and complete intoxication after one drink. The variant hasn't been pin-pointed in humans, but when it is, it will explain a lot about why some people find themselves reeling after a single drink and others can go on for hours.

The brains of alcoholics are smaller, lighter and shrunken when compared to those of nonalcoholics. Brain atrophy develops faster in women, who appear to be more sensitive than men to the cognitive consequences of alcohol use. Rat studies show that during intoxication, neurogenesis in the adult hippocampus stops in its tracks. If the rats go through detox, neurogenesis starts up again, but as long as alcohol exists in the bloodstream (even at minimal levels), neurogenesis remains on hold. In humans who suffer from chronic alcoholism, scientists hypothesize, replacement cells in the hippocampus might be absent for the better part of a lifetime. In addition, in humans, chronic alcohol abuse alters the expression of the genes that control the production of the proteins that serve as the structure of the myelin sheath, impairing function in the frontal lobes and throughout the brain.

If heavy drinkers also smoke cigarettes—and about 80 percent of alcohol-dependent individuals do—they'll experience even more acute levels of alcohol-induced brain damage, most prominently in the frontal lobes. People who smoke in midlife are nearly a third more likely to develop Alzheimer's disease than people who have never smoked. And in a study at the University of Aberdeen examining past, current and "never" smokers' skills on cognitive tests, current smokers performed significantly worse than other groups, in every capacity.

FISHING OUT THE TRUTH

When, as a child, you turned up your nose at the plate of pale fillet of sole she placed before you, your mother may have told you that fish was brain food. Plenty of studies have proven her right. As I explained in Chapter 6, there's very little that's better for your brain than the omega-3 fatty acids you get from seafood. There's a downside, of course: Exposure to the methylmercury we consume when we eat large, predatory ocean fish can result in a neurological condition that internist Jane Hightower calls "fish fog." Methylmercury does its dirty work by promoting free-radical production and inflammation in the brain—effectively speeding up the processes that cause age-related neurological decline.

Mercury is a naturally occurring element in the environment, released into the atmosphere when fossil fuels are burned. When it returns to earth, it falls into waterways and oceans, where bacteria in the water initiate chemical changes that transform mercury into methylmercury. As fish feed in these waters, they accumulate toxic chemicals. Very large, lazy fish that have done nothing all their lives but snap up smaller species carry the highest methylmercury load.

When I read the American Medical Association's resolution on mercury toxicity, I realized that maybe it was time to stop snacking on tuna sushi at lunch. More worrisome was the fact that I'd grill tuna or swordfish, or sauté halibut, for my family's dinner at least twice a week. As it turned out, these fish (the only ones my family really liked, by the way) were on the list of specimens that were dangerously high in methylmercury.

The next time I had my blood drawn, I asked my internist to order a heavy-metal panel from Quest Laboratories. As soon as I had the lab report in my hands, I could see that my level—10 micrograms per liter—was at the absolute top of the normal range. I figured that was okay.

"Mercury does not belong in the human body," Jane Hightower explained when I reported my results to her on the phone. Lab results are not very useful, she explained, because their numbers are based on occupational exposure—if you work in a factory and you have an accident with organic mercury, your level would temporarily soar. "That's not the same as having a continually elevated mercury level from the consumption of methylmercury. Ideally, the level of mercury in the blood should be zero. The Environmental Protection Agency says that a safe level is about 5 micrograms per liter, but I tell my patients that 3 micrograms is about as high as it should get." In the San Francisco area, where many people would describe themselves as fish-eating vegetarians, Hightower often sees adults with levels higher than 20 micrograms per liter. One child, a fifty-pound seven-year-old boy, had a mercury level fourteen times higher than the EPA's recommendation. He'd eaten fish twice a day for most of his life.

In *Health* magazine, journalist Ben Raines describes the case of Will Smith, a geophysicist who analyzed data for oil companies. He was having trouble functioning on the most basic levels, writes Raines. "He would leave the house for a meeting only to forget where he was going before he reached his car. Though he had lived in San Francisco for decades, he kept getting lost. And after a career spent in highly technical scientific research, the fifty-two-year-old found himself stymied by simple subtractions and unable to string words into coherent sentences." The usual diagnostic tools—tests of cardiac function, CT scans, blood work—were unrevealing. Smith's doctor told him he ought to consider finding a job that was less mentally demanding. The specialists he went to suspected encephalitis and Lou Gehrig's disease. One day, after reading the AMA's resolution, his internist phoned and asked him how much fish he ate. For years, he'd had a can of tuna as a snack three times a week, lots of sushi, especially ahi, and other kinds of fish a couple of times a week. Immediately, he abstained from fish, and in five months, because methylmercury is rapidly excreted in hair, nails, skin and feces, his symptoms had disappeared. "Stop eating fish," said Hightower, "and the fish fog goes away."

In March 2004, the Food and Drug Administration and the EPA issued a joint consumer advisory about mercury in fish and shellfish. Women who might become pregnant, nursing mothers and young children should avoid eating shark, swordfish, king mackerel or tilefish because of high levels of mercury. (For some reason, tuna, amberjack, Chilean sea bass, grouper and halibut, which have similarly high levels of mercury, were not mentioned in that advisory.) The consumer advisory suggested no restrictions for post-reproductive middle-aged folk: We could keep eating all the fish we wished, especially the "safe" species, like shrimp, canned light tuna, salmon, pollock, herring, catfish, tilapia, haddock, sardines and Pacific oysters. Confusingly, new guidelines published in 2005 from the National Oceanic and Atmospheric Administration recommended that *all* Americans eat seafood twice a week.

The EPA has a "reference dose" that says a person who weighs 100 to 154 pounds can safely ingest roughly 5 to 7 micrograms of mercury per day. That's about 1 microgram for every 22 pounds of body weight. Using those numbers, Barbara Knuth, a biological statistician at Cornell, studied mercury levels in salmon. Farmed salmon from Scotland, Norway and eastern Canada were so jam-packed with mercury, she learned, that they should be eaten no more than three times a year. Chilean farmed salmon was safe for six dinners annually. Wild salmon—pink, sockeye and coho—were acceptable table fodder twice a month. Wild chum salmon—which is the hardest to come by, unless you do the fishing yourself—was okay for one meal a week.

If you are eating one of the fish known to have high levels of methyl-mercury—say, ahi tuna—the EPA's reference dose means that you can have about an eighth of a pound, not much more than a single order of sushi. A survey of top California sushi restaurants showed that the mercury level in tuna was on average double the FDA limit—so you might want to restrict your intake to a single piece of tuna maki.

Americans eat about one billion pounds of canned and "pouched" tuna annually, which makes it big business. I'd eagerly embraced the rumor that it was low in mercury (which I now admit did not make much sense since it came from a large, lazy fish) and was enjoying regular tuna-relish-mayonnaise sandwiches until I read that a scientist on the FDA's food-advisory committee had personally tested ten cans of tuna for mercury. He found that one brand contained 1.24 parts per million of mercury, more than 500 percent the FDA's published average for canned tuna, so high in fact that FDA regulations of 480 micrograms of methylmercury in a pound of fish would prevent the sale of it to the public. That's enough to make you give up tuna melts forever, but there's help on the way. Recently, in my local supermarket, I noticed a sign on the ice in the fresh fish display case for Safe Harbor Certified Seafood. Further research revealed that Safe Harbor was the brainchild of Micro Analytical Systems, a company founded in 2002 to develop technology for analyzing the purity of foods. I flashed on the image of the fish guy at Whole Foods testing my tilapia, but more practically, the fish are analyzed at the wholesaler's before they're shipped to the market. Testers extract a sample of flesh with a syringe and a biopsy needle, and insert it into a device about the size of a copy machine. It takes about a minute to analyze a sample. According to Malcolm Wittenberg, the company's CEO, at least half the fish tested for mercury content are rejected. Only those with mercury levels well below the FDA's recommended level make the cut.

THE TOXIC LOAD

Your memory impairment may have more to do with your job than you ever suspected. If you work in a new building, constructed with energy-efficient insulation materials, and you can't open your windows, chances are good that you're getting too much carbon monoxide and not enough fresh air. Carbon monoxide poisoning need not be acute. It can occur even when small amounts are inhaled over a long time, for instance in an office with poor ventilation. As carbon monoxide is inhaled, it enters the bloodstream and attaches to hemoglobin, the blood protein that carries oxygen to the hippocampus, causing neurons to lose vitality and eventually die. A $60 investment in two carbon monoxide detectors, one for the office and one for the home, can provide you with everything you need to know about your exposure.

We don't go out of our way to ingest toxic chemicals, but it happens every day. When I moved from New York to Los Angeles in the late 1980s, I discovered that gardening, a pursuit I'd enjoyed during brief New England summers, was a competitive sport in our neighborhood of bungalows. No longer was it sufficient to grow a springtime passel of peonies and then harvest a bumper crop of tomatoes and zukes in August. Gardening in southern California was more like exterior decorating, except that it went on fifty-two weeks a year. Of course, everything was subject to pestilent invasion—aphids clung to the roses, snails devoured the primroses, caterpillars ate up the sweet peas. Once a month, the mow-blow-and-go crew of gardeners altered their normal thirty-minute routine and strapped on backpacks equipped with canisters filled with pesticides and herbicides.

Where the gardeners left off, the exterminators took over. They arrived quarterly, spraying everything in sight—the cracks where house and driveway met, the window frames, and inside the house, the baseboards and grout around the tub. My husband assured me that this was the way it was done in southern California, and that I did not want to become familiar with the creatures that would join us if spraying ceased. Besides the cockroaches, ants and rodents, there would be spiders, he said darkly. These were not the daddy longlegs I knew from New England picnics. Indeed, in our alley, overrun with bougainvillea and ivy, I'd seen a couple of scurrying, bulked-up, furry arachnids.

I could always tell when the sprayers had visited us. The air inside and out reeked of chemicals, smelling something like petroleum, but with a sweetish note that made it all the more disgusting. I'd leave immediately, but within minutes of exposure, my eyes burned, my stomach churned, and my throat closed up. I felt dizzy and distracted. My head ached, and over half a decade, I developed a reverberating bronchial hack, which made people sidle away from me at cocktail parties. It didn't help that, in the name of pest protection, the dog and cat wore flea collars and had occasional flea dips. When things got really itchy, we sprinkled their beds (and when they cuddled up, they sprinkled ours) with flea powder.

Don't ask me why, but I never attributed my symptoms to what was being sprayed in and around my house. I chalked all of them up—the hack, the headaches, the dizziness—to air pollution, which is something you live with when you live in Los Angeles. By the time I'd been in the southland for ten years, I'd begun to have extreme reactions not only to pesticides, but also to hair sprays, cigarettes, gasoline, air fresheners, fabric dyes, perfumes, soaps, enamel paint and oven cleaner. The first floor of a department store was an eye-stinging, headache-provoking maze, to be navigated as quickly as possible. I bought and returned a Tempur-Pedic bed pillow because I could not tolerate its acrid odor. The same was true of the wrist rest I purchased for my keyboard: To me, it reeked. Nobody else could smell a thing.

Not until we moved the family to northern California, where people pick the aphids off their roses rather than dousing them in pesticides, did it occur to me that I'd been living in a toxic sea of chlorpyrifos, an organophosphate that affects the nervous system in much the same way as nerve gas. Absorbed by the skin, mucous membranes, gastrointestinal tract and lungs, organophosphate pesticides produce symptoms of memory loss, sleep disturbance and depression, as well as immune dysfunction resulting in chronic fatigue syndrome, fibromyalgia and chronic asthma. When organophosphates reach toxic levels, they block the breakdown of the neurotransmitter acetylcholine, interfering with the transmission of nerve signals in the brains of insects, rodents, pets and humans alike. In insects and rodents, organophosphates inhibit acetylcholine breakdown to such a degree that it accumulates in the neuromuscular junction and impedes the function of the diaphragm, resulting in suffocation. In addition to blocking the breakdown of acetylcholine by inhibiting acetylcholinesterase, organophosphates (and for that matter, most toxins) cause oxidative damage to cells, launching the cycle I described in Chapter 6. Some people possess genes that predispose them to sensitivity to chemical agents, particularly those in agricultural pesticides. I suspected, but couldn't prove, that I was one of the genetically susceptible.

Within a few weeks of the move north, many of my symptoms, including the hacking asthmatic cough, went away. My memory didn't improve, and I was still highly sensitive to these toxins. I'd have to be careful, for the rest of my life. On a June camping trip to the Sierra Nevada mountain range, where mosquitoes were rife, I applied OFF! Deep Woods, with a concentration of 23.9 percent DEET, guaranteed to last for three to five hours. Within two hours, the insects were landing on me, so I sprayed my hiking shirt and shorts. Within twenty minutes, I thought I had the flu. I was woozy, headachy, and thoroughly disoriented. It might have been the double dose of DEET, or the fact that I was also taking an antihistamine, with similar inhibitory effects on the breakdown of acetylcholine, but the fact was, I didn't feel any better until I strung up the "solar shower," a two-and-a-half-gallon bag of slightly warm water, and scrubbed the OFF! off. Needless to say, the mosquitoes had a field day.

The more I looked, the more I found. Much of the cognitive impairment we attributed to age-related memory deficits, or incipient Alzheimer's disease, actually had other antecedents.

15

WHAT YOUR DOCTOR
FORGOT TO TELL YOU
• • •
Prescription Drugs and "Safe" Over-the-Counter Meds

May Account for Your Fogginess

Your physician may be unaware that the drugs you're taking are making you as foggy as a summer's day in San Francisco. In most cases the FDA does not require cognitive side effects to be mentioned in product literature or advertising, so there's very little incentive for pharmaceutical companies to spend money on research that certainly won't boost sales. Even when physicians are aware of the cognitive implications of the drugs they prescribe, these may reasonably take a backseat to other priorities, such as keeping you alive.

Jack, a veterinarian, had a heart attack and multiple bypass surgery at the age of forty-six. Among his many prescriptions were Inderal, an antihypertensive beta-blocker, and Lozol, a diuretic. "In all the years I've been taking those drugs," he said, "not one doctor has ever mentioned memory loss to me." He'd actually looked up Inderal in the *Physician's Desk Reference* a few weeks earlier, just out of curiosity, and there it was, big as day, under adverse side effects: "short-term memory loss." In other words, it's a known treatment-related adverse effect. "I suspect I've been suffering for years," he said, "and I never heard a thing about it." These medications were key to his cardiac health, so he couldn't stop taking them. But just knowing what they did brought some relief. "When I have memory issues, I'm no longer going to assume that it's age or incipient Alzheimer's disease. It helps to be able to put my memory lapses in perspective."

As drug molecules move through the bloodstream, they experience their own form of Vessel Identity Syndrome. They encounter neural receptors that vaguely resemble their identified targets and agreeably hitch up with them, provoking all sorts of cognitive shenanigans.

Much of the trouble arises when people fail to follow instructions. Especially with over-the-counter drugs, they adopt the "more must be better" tactic. With prescription drugs, they fall back on the "Oops, I forgot, so I'll double up" approach, a surefire way to engender drug-related cognitive side effects.

Among the drugs likely to cause you problems: anti-anxiety drugs and antidepressants, sedatives and hypnotics, antacids, antihistamines, corticosteriods, beta-blockers, cough medicines, diuretics and chemotherapy, as well as drugs to prevent incontinence, ulcers, elevated cholesterol and diabetes. As I discovered a dozen years ago, drugs intended to prevent motion sickness are also capable of snatching away your memory.

Some years ago, in preparation for a trip to the Pacific Northwest, I asked my doctor for a Transderm Scop—a motion-sickness patch that I thought would get me through the ferry ride from Seattle to Vancouver. With my four-year-old son along, I couldn't afford to wind up hanging over the rail. Before embarking, I pressed the patch behind my ear as directed, found us good seats, and prepared for a long and scenic ride. That's the last thing I remember. In less than ten minutes, I had sunk into helpless sleep, the kind where your mouth hangs open and you drool.

When I woke up two hours later, it took several seconds for me to understand that I was on a big boat, and a few panicky minutes to find my kid, who was enjoying the wonders of aerosol-propelled Cheez Whiz on crackers. He was playing a game of old maid with three children whose parents were wide awake and shocked by my behavior. Still feeling like I was trying to climb out of a bucket of wet sand, I pointed to the flesh-colored patch on my neck. Then I walked my boy out to the deck for some fresh air. Apparently, a pod of orcas leapt to the surface as we approached the rail. The truth is, I don't remember a thing.

It was frustrating and scary, but also galvanizing. Why on earth would a doctor give me a drug with such memory-obliterating consequences? I'd asked for it, certainly, but wasn't it his job to inform me of the side effects?

"Not really," he said, when I called to tell him what had happened. "If I were to mention every possible adverse reaction that any patient might have to any drug . . . well, that would be impossible."

I discovered that drugs given for motion sickness—the scopolamine transdermal patch, or its older cousins, Dramamine and Bonine—are notorious for inducing temporary amnesia. These drugs (and many others) work by preventing the release of acetylcholine, which regulates activity in the hippocampus.

Drugs that block the production or uptake of acetylcholine are referred to as "anticholinergics," and there are many of them on the market. They give you desert mouth and blurred vision and make you sleepy. They cause impairments in learning and memory storage, in attention and speed of processing.

The anesthesia you receive during surgery or during long and painful dental procedures also has powerful anticholinergic properties—in fact, that's the whole idea. If you were given only painkillers, you wouldn't feel a thing, but you'd recall, to your everlasting detriment, what it looked, smelled and sounded like when the surgeon unzipped your abdomen or sawed your tooth in half. As you age, the drugs used to anesthetize you, usually some combination of nitrous oxide, ketamine and isoflurane, become increasingly obliterative, especially if you're unconscious for a prolonged period. These drugs sometimes produce both anterograde amnesia—a lack of memory of what occurred before the surgery—and retrograde amnesia, an absence of recollection of what occurred after they wheeled you into the recovery room. One of the survey respondents, who'd undergone spinal surgery, noted that, from his bed on the day after his operation, he'd ordered several pieces of computer equipment. When they arrived at his house barely forty-eight hours later, he'd answered the door and sworn to the UPS driver that Best Buy must have made a big mistake.

MAGICAL MEMORY THIEVES

Diphenhydramine, the active ingredient in Benadryl and some other over-the-counter allergy medicines, as well as the sleep inducer in Tylenol PM, will reliably diminish your cognitive abilities. "I rely a lot on Benadryl for sleep and allergy control," remarked Leslie. "I take it almost every night." She'd just finished telling me that she couldn't figure out why it was so hard to haul herself out of bed in the morning, or why she felt foggy until noon. A study at the University of Iowa found that diphenhydramine caused more driving impairment than being legally drunk, I told her.

It ought to go without saying that it's a bad idea to use "nighttime" cold medicines (laden with diphenhydramine) during the day, but people do it. Not long ago, I stood in a long line at the local shipping and packing store, while the painfully slow clerk explained to each customer that he had a terrible cold, and had been hitting the Nyquil hard, a practice he described as "Quillin' it day and night." When my package went astray, having been posted by him to New Jersey instead of New York, I wasn't surprised.

Some drugs that suppress stomach acid are also anticholinergic. Too much Pepcid or Zantac and you won't be able to remember what it was that you ate. Prevacid and Nexium do not appear to have cognitive side effects.

Despite their claims to the contrary, the newer "nondrowsy" allergy medicines like Claritin, Allegra and Zyrtec can make you very sleepy: In one clinical trial, 14 percent of Zyrtec users experienced drowsiness. On the other hand, individuals with allergic rhinitis consistently exhibit significant declines in cognitive processing, psychomotor speed, verbal learning and memory during allergy season. Whether you take allergy medications or do without them, you may wind up like my Boston cabdriver, who was sneezing so hard when he collected me for a springtime trip to the airport that I thought we'd have an accident on Memorial Drive. When I suggested that an inherent aspect of sneezing—closing your eyes—was perhaps not safe at fifty miles per hour in heavy traffic, he agreed. He'd tried all the allergy medications, he said, "but they knock me out. I'm not alert, I had a couple of near misses, and I can't remember how to get where I'm going."

Corticosteroids, such as prednisone, are another class of drugs that do your memory no favors. Used to treat asthma, arthritis, allergies and pain, they impair long-term memory as well as immediate recall by overwhelming the hippocampus with cortisol. (When researchers want to induce memory loss in rodents, they inject them with corticosteroids.) Despite plenty of studies that demonstrate cortisone's amnesiac effects, physicians love to prescribe these drugs, mostly because they work like magic. My son's ear, nose and throat doctor told us that he could get rid of both of our pollen allergies before breakfast the next day by giving each of us an injection of cortisone. But what about memory? I asked. What about the effect on the hippocampus? He shrugged. He'd given at least ten thousand of these injections during his career, without a bit of trouble. "Maybe that's because your patients don't attribute their forgetfulness to your shots," I said snarkily. He shrugged. "It's better than sneezing for four months straight," he said.

Kristin, an executive and the mother of three, took prednisone, a corticosteroid, to calm down an allergy to sunscreen. Normally fairly well-organized, in one month she reported that she lost track of her wallet three times, as well as her laptop, her cell phone, purse, keys and sunglasses. "Three times, they called me from Safeway to come get my red wallet, because I'd left it in the cart," she said. "I had renewed faith in humankind by the time the month of treatment was over and my head returned to my shoulders."

As Jack, the veterinarian, discovered, antihypertensive drugs, both beta-blockers (Inderal and Lopressor) and other blood-pressure medications (Aldoclor, Aldomet and Aldoril), can induce forgetfulness. They are prescribed to lower blood pressure, as well as for other indications, and have been reported in clinical investigations to produce cognitive side effects, including memory loss and impairment of verbal memory. Peggy, the corporate consultant, revealed that for years she'd been taking Inderal for an off-label indication—to prevent migraines. After years of excruciating pain, the drug had saved her, but her doctor had never mentioned that Inderal affected the ability to consolidate short-term memory.

Oxybutynin chloride—the "overactive bladder" medication that many midlife women use—is a powerfully anticholinergic memory killer. Diuretics, often used to reduce premenstrual bloating, have a similar effect. Your doctor didn't mention that? Why am I not surprised?

CHEMOTHERAPY DRUGS

For decades, chemotherapy patients who complained of memory problems were told that their difficulties resulted from depression, anxiety or the treatment-related ovarian failure. Recently, in brain-imaging studies, researchers observed that in some women, the chemo-treated brain looked twenty-five years older than it actually was. There was also a reduction of metabolic activity in the parts of the brain involving language. According to an article in the *Wall Street Journal*, studies of breast cancer patients showed that nearly two-thirds of women treated with chemotherapy developed some level of cognitive problems, though most recovered over weeks or months. About a quarter developed problems that never went away. Andrew Saykin, at Dartmouth Medical School, suggests that the neurotoxic effects of chemotherapy might lead to atrophy of cerebral gray matter and the eventual destruction of the myelin sheath that protects the nerves and allows for uninterrupted transmission of nerve impulses.

"The doctors talk about everything else—the nausea, the hair loss—but I guess they think that memory loss is too insignificant to bother with," said Katya, who underwent months of chemotherapy before and after stem cell replacement. "I've had to piece together what has happened in my life. For a long time, I felt like a stranger in my own house and neighborhood. It's a small price to pay, of course, for being alive. But it does bad things to your self-esteem; you already feel like you're helpless, and not being able to remember anything just proves the point. It could've been the chemo that wiped me out, but I was taking so many drugs, including Ativan for anxiety and queasiness, Zantac and Prilosec [the stomach acid suppressors] and a huge amount of Benadryl to help with the allergic reaction to the chemo drugs. For a long time it was paralyzing—sort of a semiconscious nightmare, where you have to consciously piece together what is happening in your life. I screwed up every appointment I had. I'd forget where I was, in territory where I've driven my whole adult life, and have to pull off the road and call someone familiar with the area to get my bearings. My friends bore the brunt of this. I crapped out on people all the time. I'd make plans and completely forget they existed."

PLAYING WITH GABA

Psychiatric medications (antidepressants and anti-anxiety drugs) and hypnotic sedatives (sleeping pills) are among the most commonly used cognition-impairing pharmaceuticals. Often people take more than one mood-enhancing drug at a time, compounding the problem. Benzodiazepines, the drugs that doctors prescribe to reduce anxiety, include Ativan, Xanax, Halcion, Restoril and Valium. Introduced in the early 1960s, these drugs replaced barbiturates, on which people overdosed easily and often. By 1979, one in five women and one in ten men were on benzos, which work by enhancing the action of the inhibitory neurotransmitter GABA, which slows synaptic communication and produces a markedly impaired ability to absorb new information. For people suffering from serious anxiety problems, these drugs provide immediate relief, but, said Richard Friedman, the director of psychopharmacology at New York Hospital, "they definitely affect working memory. Their primary clinical effect is to induce sedation. They have enormous potential for abuse and addiction."

The drugs are vastly overprescribed, he added. "They may be useful at the beginning, like pain medication for a broken leg, but at least 30 percent of the people who come to see me have been taking them long-term." A very prominent publisher told Friedman that he was having terrible memory problems, so extreme that he didn't want to meet people or engage in conversation—it was too embarrassing. It turned out that he'd been on Ativan for twenty-five years. "He didn't know why he was on it," Friedman said. "It was a habit. When he came off, his memory came back."

Earlier generations of antidepressant drugs, including Elavil, a popular tricyclic, were acknowledged as flagrant hijackers of memory. But today's SSRIs (and a newer category called SNRIs) can also make some people feel as dull as an old linoleum floor. The novelist John Irving stopped taking the drugs after concluding that they made him feel detached and dulled his urge to write. Charles Nemeroff, chairman of psychiatry and behavioral sciences at Emory University, estimates that between 15 and 20 percent of his patients complain that they feel blunted on the drugs. No one's proved it, but scientists suspect that serotonin-based antidepressants sneak into dopamine receptors, displacing their rightful occupants, the dopamine neurotransmitters that are critical to frontal-lobe function. You feel better as the brain begins to produce increased BDNF and new cells in the hippocampus flourish, but without sufficient dopamine in circulation, you lose the inclination to sit up and pay attention, and the world passes you by in a blur. Even without supplementary serotonin, dopamine levels take a nosedive as you age. In each decade of adult life, a specific receptor for dopamine—the one that acts as a welcoming committee for the chemical, drawing it deep within the cell—declines by 6 to 7 percent.

As dopamine receptors diminish in number, writes Nora Volkow, a scientist at the Brookhaven National Laboratory, so does the ability to problem-solve, think abstractly and carry out multiple tasks simultaneously.

One woman in her late forties, who had taken Paxil for ten years, observed that she'd failed several college courses recently, despite dedicating forty hours a week to homework and studying. "I was frequently an honor roll student in high school, with a super-strong, almost photographic visual memory. Nothing seems to stick anymore, and I flunked all my tests." She wasn't suffering from depression, she said—in fact, she'd been fine since her divorce, seven years before. She stayed on the drugs as a preventive measure, she explained—just in case something else went awry.

Don't get me wrong: For individuals with specific types of recurring psychiatric problems, including major depressive disorder, when these drugs are effective, they're invaluable. For other patients, those who suffer from occasional mild depression, or who experience distress over specific events, such as divorce, illness or a death in the family, the drugs, taken for an extended period, may be more debilitating than the original bout with the blues. The brain is a highly integrated organ, observes Peter Breggin, who opposes the "quick and dirty" prescribing of antidepressants, especially for long-term use. "Emotional suffering cannot be dulled," he explained, "without harming other functions, such as concentration, alertness, sensitivity and self-awareness."

In Chapter 13, I observed that sleeping pills didn't work for chronic insomniacs. On the other hand, for people who have occasional difficulties getting to sleep, non-benzo hypnotics, such as Ambien and Sonata, can help. Like benzodiazepines, these drugs act on the neurotransmitter GABA. They link up with the cell-surface structures known as GABA receptors, and kick them into high gear, slowing down your central nervous system so much that it is impossible for you to stay awake. In theory, non-benzo hypnotics do not affect sleep architecture. In practice, it's another story. "You look at the polysomnography," says Michael Perlis, a sleep researcher at the University of

Rochester, "and you can easily see that there's a difference, in slow-wave sleep and in REM." The newer hypnotics have fewer cognitive side effects than their benzodiazepine cousins. Still, for some, they have amnesic properties that can get you in serious trouble if you're not safely tucked under the covers within minutes of swallowing a tablet.

There is a warning taped on the vial of every Ambien prescription, and lately, there's also a directive on the product literature: "Once you take this drug, get directly into bed and go to sleep, and be prepared to sleep a full night." Apparently, enough people have discovered the repercussions of not going straight to bed to make the warning necessary. Ambien and Sonata both have a short half-life, which means that you may wake up in the middle of the night and do some strange things.

"I took Ambien almost nightly for six weeks, which of course was longer than you're supposed to—seven to ten days is what the directions say, but my doctor told me it was okay, that the drug would continue to be effective. I woke up a couple of times to the remnants of meals I do not remember eating," writes Lisbeth. "I hid money, and did not find it until I ripped my house apart. I canceled an appointment and changed another appointment without remembering that I did it."

An entire message board on the Internet is devoted to comments from people who have had zombie-type experiences on Ambien, some of which are vaguely amusing—nonsensical conversations with confused bedmates, for instance—and others, including car accidents and leaving the stove on, that are obviously very dangerous. Some people reported that these amnesic experiences continued well into the next day, leaving them with big gaps in their recollections. "I find my daytime memory seriously affected," wrote Jana. "I've set up the coffee-pot and forgotten to put coffee in it. I've forgotten whether I took my other meds, and I've left ingredients out of things I'm cooking. No big deal in themselves, but multiplied many times a day, very alarming. I feel like I've killed some 'connect the dots' brain cells."

As I noted previously, a new generation of sleep-enhancing pharmaceuticals intended to increase quality rather than quantity of sleep is in the works. We won't see those for a while, but tweaked versions of non-benzo hypnotics are already available. Ambien CR, a slow-release formula, will likely prevent people from waking up in the middle of the night and messily raiding the refrigerator. After a six-month clinical trial, Lunesta, the longer-acting sleep medicine (plan on eight full hours) that Sepracor launched in 2005, received FDA approval for extended use. The commercial caught my eye: Lunesta's long-term efficacy made it useful for the treatment of chronic insomnia.

Despite the fact that I'd had terrible experiences with Ambien and Sonata, I wanted to test Lunesta. I called my internist and told her that work had been keeping me up nights: My mind was an amusement park of whirling, spinning words, and they wouldn't let me sleep. As if I was ordering at a drive-in window of Wendy's, I told her what I wanted—Lunesta, in the 2-milligram dose. I was not to take it for more than two weeks, she cautioned, and I promised that I would not. The first night was fine—I sacked out for eight hours, and woke up feeling as refreshed as the people in the TV commercials. That morning, in front of the computer monitor, I inspected my brain for telltale signs of fogginess. I couldn't find any. In fact, I felt terrific: I'd had two more hours of sleep than I usually got. Three days later—when Ambien always cut out on me—Lunesta was still working. Ten days later, I was still sleeping through eight-hour nights.

Then, it was time to toast a friend's fiftieth birthday. Alcohol (because of its GABA-enhancing properties) is strictly forbidden with Lunesta, and I wanted a glass of wine. Declaring the experiment a success, I decided that it was time to quit. I waited for the nasty rebound insomnia that can arise when GABA is no longer artificially enhanced. The first night, I was a little bit restless, which was hardly unusual. The second night, I slept fine, with a single brief awakening at 4:00 A.M.

I found that my attitude toward sleep had undergone a subtle shift. No longer was it a teasing lover: I could have it whenever I wanted it. Was it possible that I could train myself to sleep for two more hours every night by judiciously using Lunesta to reset my circadian rhythms? I put it on the list of things I intended to discuss with Tracy Kuo on my next trip to Stanford. At the very least, she'd be amused: On my last visit I'd told her in no uncertain terms that I'd never again use a hypnotic sedative because I hated the cognitive side effects. How satisfying it would be, I thought, if I could take a pharmaceutical that everyone agreed could cause cognitive impairment, and turn it to my advantage.

16

THE LAST PLACE YOU LOOK

. . .

Thyroid Low? Blood Pressure High?
A Host of Common Midlife Disorders
Pack a Cognitive Wallop

Cognitive impairment often accompanies such grave patholo-gies as diabetes, lupus, Parkinson's syndrome, multiple sclero-sis, epilepsy and Cushing's disease. But a host of other disorders also result in deficits in memory and attention. Your doctor may tell you that it's nothing, just age-related cognitive decline—or that it's seri-ous, the onset of Alzheimer's disease—when something else entirely is going on.

Amy Tan, author of *The Joy Luck Club* and *The Kitchen God's Wife,* suffered for nearly five years from Lyme disease before a hema-tologist who specializes in tick-borne diseases pinpointed the cause of her cognitive problems. Her internist and multiple neurologists were stumped. They ordered an MRI, and discovered fifteen lesions in her brain, in the frontal and medial temporal lobes. Her father, sister and brother had died of brain tumors, and her mother had recently passed away after a struggle with Alzheimer's. The doctors' presumption, Tan said, and hers was that she was in the grip of an unidentified dementing disease. "I couldn't think with it, and I couldn't write. And I really had no idea of what was going on for about four years. . . . When you have this terrorist in your body, you don't have control."

She never noticed the telltale bull's-eye rash that is the mark of Lyme disease. Nor does she recall developing the associated flulike symptoms. She thought that whatever had overtaken her body and mind would end her career. (It didn't: She published a collection of nonfiction essays, *The Opposite of Fate*, one of which details her experience with Lyme disease.) She felt like she was hanging on, word by word. Her husband observed that her mind was becoming disorganized; as she grew weaker, he had to do almost everything for her. Eventually, Tan found a reference on the Internet to the neurological symptoms of late-stage Lyme disease and found her way to Raphael Stricker, a San Francisco hematologist who treats tick-borne diseases. A protracted course of antibiotics helped with other symptoms, but the neurological deficits appear to be hers for life. If she'd been diagnosed and treated in a timely fashion, she never would have experienced them.

Just as vexing, and at least as difficult to diagnose, chronic fatigue syndrome causes debilitating exhaustion, vertigo, low-grade fever, severe insomnia, muscle aches and brain fog. Recently, scientists identified a likely trigger in this poorly understood disorder (frequently mistaken for hypochondria or depression), which affects nearly a million people and can emerge at the tail end of a viral infection. In the spring of 2006, a ground-breaking Centers for Disease Control and Prevention study of chronic fatigue syndrome revealed differences in genes relevant to the immune system and the sympathetic nervous system. Among them were slightly abnormal genes that regulate the HPA axis. Researchers postulate that chronic fatigue syndrome represents a genetically mediated over-the-top response to very mild physical or emotional stress. In three to five years, there should be a diagnostic test—and treatment.

Certainly, not all "missed" diagnoses and explanations have such severe consequences. Still, it's good to know what you're up against. Two examples: Cognitive dysfunction, known as "pump head," that lasts for six months to a year is a common complication of cardiopulmonary bypass surgery, affecting a fifth of patients who have been placed on a cardiac pump. But no one tells the patients. "My cardiologist never mentioned it to me, and neither did my surgeon," said Justin, an attorney for a nonprofit organization who had a triple bypass. "I'm not sure that they're interested in your brain—it's really low in their priorities. But I was foggy—just really feeling dumb—for so long that it wasn't clear that I could keep going to work. We thought it was Alzheimer's disease. I would have been better off if someone had just clued me in."

Doctors have been known to diagnose a stroke, when the actual problem involves your sex life. It's rare—affecting fewer than 25 out of 100,000 people each year—but if you develop transient global amnesia, where you can't remember what happened in the last six to twelve hours and new memories are not sticking, consider the possibility that you may have executed what is known as "the Valsalva maneuver" with too much enthusiasm. Bearing down hard, as some people do during sex, while snow shoveling or, for that matter, when having a bowel movement, creates intense pressure on the brain's blood vessels, resulting in temporary lack of blood flow to the temporal lobes. Memories of the hours just before, during and after are gone forever, and the afflicted individual may also lose recall of events that occurred days, weeks or months earlier.

OBESITY, GLUCOSE AND INSULIN

Until a few years ago, scientists thought the brain sat in a privileged position. No matter what occurred in the body, it would get what it needed. That's not the case. Often, the brain is the last in line. Other tissues can make use of amino acids, but for the brain, it's glucose or bust.

When your doctor tells you that you need to keep an eye on your waistline or drop ten pounds, there's usually a discussion of the risk of coronary heart disease. The cognitive risk is equally significant, but it's rarely mentioned, said UCSF researcher Kristine Yaffe, because "your average physician is not thinking that if someone is fat, it may affect [his] brain." Two-thirds of American men are overweight. So are more than 50 percent of American women. Usually, too many pounds are accompanied by "metabolic syndrome," a group of risk factors that includes excessive fat tissue in and around the abdomen (the classic "pot belly"), high cholesterol levels, elevated blood pressure and elevated high-sensitivity C-reactive protein in the blood, indicating inflammation. New studies show that metabolic syndrome significantly speeds the rate of cognitive decline and dramatically increases the probability of developing Alzheimer's disease.

Putting on the pounds is the first step toward developing a condition that scientists, depending on their perspective, refer to as insulin resistance or impaired glucose tolerance.

At the heart of the problem is the body's ability to handle glucose, or blood sugar. To keep things running smoothly physiologically, the level of glucose in the blood must remain within the range of 70 to 100 milligrams per 100 milliliters. For more than 40 percent of U.S. adults over forty years old, blood glucose levels are too high, making the pancreas, which produces insulin, work far too hard. Insulin acts as a key, unlocking receptors that drag glucose out of the bloodstream and into the cell, where it can be processed into energy. When you're insulin resistant (or have impaired glucose tolerance), insulin can't open the gates. Glucose remains in the bloodstream. And as long as glucose is in the bloodstream, the pancreas doesn't receive the signal that immediate needs for insulin have been satisfied. Instead of shutting down the works, it keeps making more insulin. The brain, which, as you know, utilizes glucose as its primary fuel, finds itself seriously shortchanged, and recognizes the glucose shortage as the worst kind of stress. The cells of the sensitive hippocampus suffer, cutting down on the production of BDNF, as well as the production of neurotransmitters required for memory. To make it worse, the glucose left coursing through the bloodstream gets stored as fat, mostly around your middle.

Antonio Convit, a researcher at New York University, studies impaired glucose tolerance and its relationship to cognitive dysfunction. There are no symptoms of impaired glucose tolerance, he told me. You can't tell if you have it. It has nothing to do with that lightheaded feeling you get when you don't eat enough. It's relatively easy to test for it, however. You need a glucose tolerance test, which should not be confused with the glucose test that your doctor orders when he sends you for a CBC panel as part of your physical exam. The glucose tolerance test requires an overnight fast, followed by an early morning blood test. Then, on an empty stomach, you drink a beverage with 75 grams of sugar in it. Two hours later, you have another blood test. If the value of that test is under 140, you have normal glucose tolerance. If it's between 140 and 200, you have impaired glucose tolerance. If it's over 200, you are one of the seventeen million people in the United States who have type 2 diabetes.

People who have impaired glucose tolerance—shockingly, that's nearly half of the adult U.S. population—are often on their way to developing type 2 diabetes, with its accompanying risks of hypertension, heart attack and stroke, Convit explained. According to the *New York Times*, forty-one million people in the United States are prediabetic, and epidemiologists predict that one in three American children born in 2000 will eventually develop type 2 diabetes. Long before diabetes shows up, cognitive deficits will be evident. "The higher the level of blood sugar in the body," Convit noted when I interviewed him, "the worse a person performs on memory tests of delayed and immediate recall." In brain scans, Convit found that the hippocampi of subjects with impaired glucose tolerance were significantly smaller than those of patients with normal levels.

The good news, said Convit, is that impaired glucose tolerance is relatively easy to fix. "Lose weight," he explained, "about 10 percent of your body mass, and take up strength exercise in the form of light weight and resistance training, and in most cases, glucose levels will return to normal, and the cognitive problems will resolve."

For most people, 10 percent of body mass is well under twenty-five pounds. Training with light weights, several days a week, doesn't even require a trip to the gym. So why would impaired glucose tolerance continue to be a problem for a large percentage of the population? There are no equivalent statistics for women, but two-thirds of American men (in addition to being overweight) are not regularly active. One-quarter do not participate in any physical activity at all. As obesity rates climb, impaired glucose tolerance is showing up in people in their teens and twenties, which suggests that by the time they're middle-aged, they may experience a substantial decline in cognitive function. "We're hoping that recognizing the implications for the brain," Convit explained, "will galvanize into action people who otherwise wouldn't start exercising and shed the extra pounds."

Roger, the retired air-traffic controller you met in Chapter 2, has all the risk factors for metabolic syndrome. He's had a significant weight problem since he was eight years old. But until last year, no doctor informed him that his obesity, elevated cholesterol and high blood pressure likely triggered the cognitive problems that eventually compelled him to leave his high-pressure job. "To be honest, I didn't struggle with my weight," Roger told me. "I was okay with it. I ate what I wanted to eat, which was a lot, and took the meds the doctors gave me, figuring they would keep things in check. I didn't realize that my elevated glucose levels were wrecking my memory." In the six months after Roger heard the news about metabolic syndrome, he lost eighty-five pounds. He plans to lose another twenty. "My glucose levels are approaching more normal numbers," he told me. "But wouldn't it be the pits if the cheesecake and Häagen-Dazs I enjoyed so much accelerated my mental decline?"

There are reasons to drop the pounds and pick up the weights that go far beyond midlife forgetfulness. At the University of Washington, researcher Suzanne Craft hypothesizes that when insulin is poorly controlled over a period of time, this may trigger a series of reactions in the brain that lead to the development of Alzheimer's disease. In this chain reaction, insulin resistance (Craft's preferred description of the body's inability to draw glucose into the cells) triggers elevations of proteins that are similar to those found in the plaques of the brains of individuals with Alzheimer's. Long-term insulin resistance is also associated with higher levels of inflammation of the central nervous system. The combination of elevated brain proteins and inflammation may be an important risk factor for the development of the disease.

HYPERTENSION

Chronic hypertension, otherwise known as high blood pressure, is also associated with a measurable decline in cognitive function on a broad range of tasks. Once again, there are no telltale signs. It's closely associated with obesity, but many normal-weight or thin people are also hypertensive. Over 20 percent of adult Americans suffer from it—and one-third of them, the ones who don't have regular physicals, don't know it. Normal blood pressure is 120/80. Hypertension is defined as a systolic reading (the top number) of over 140, and a diastolic reading (the bottom number) of over 90. Doctors start issuing warnings around 130/85, but in truth, they should address the problem as soon as it is evident that blood pressure is starting to climb. The borderline reading you get in the doctor's office by no means tells the whole story: What counts cognitively is whether your blood pressure dips 10 to 20 percent, as it's supposed to, when you lie down at night. If your blood pressure is borderline, your physician should order a reading with an ambulatory blood pressure monitor, about the size of a pack of cards, with a small cuff that checks your blood pressure every thirty minutes. It won't take long to find out what your blood pressure is doing when you're not in the doctor's office. If you're slipping over the line, you want to take action immediately. Borderline hypertension responds quickly to increased amounts of aerobic exercise. The sooner you find out about it, the better chance you have of preserving your brain.

IN YOUR BLOOD

Under ideal conditions, the body replaces old red blood cells by making about two million new ones per second. Those new blood cells are great at hooking up with oxygen and delivering it when and where it is needed in the body. Anemia is a blood condition identified by a lower-than-normal number of red blood cells, usually measured by a decrease in the amount of hemoglobin. Hemoglobin is the red pigment in red blood cells that transports oxygen throughout the body. When you're anemic, hemoglobin molecules are in short supply and insufficient oxygen reaches the brain, resulting in exhaustion, pallor, loss of muscle strength and cognitive deficits. It's quite common—12 percent of premenopausal women are anemic, as are 13 percent of people over seventy. No figures exist for middle-aged people, but physicians mistake anemia for a host of other problems, diagnosing depression, chronic fatigue syndrome and Alzheimer's disease. Risk factors for anemia include heavy menstrual periods, pregnancy and older age, as well as serious diseases that cause anemia such as chronic kidney disease, diabetes, heart disease, cancer, rheumatoid arthritis, inflammatory bowel disease and HIV. Doses of highly oxidative supplemental iron are no longer prescribed. Increased quantities of red meats, egg yolks, beans, fish, poultry and whole grain bread usually do the trick. In older people, the deficit often results from insufficient levels of vitamin B-12 and folic acid, both of which are required for the production of new red blood cells.

SUBCLINICAL HYPOTHYROIDISM

Sometimes, what you suspect is true in the beginning turns out to be right after all. Several years before I thought of writing this book, but soon after my family moved to northern California, I took a long look at myself. I was forty-two. I was so tired and thin that you would have thought I'd carried the moving boxes up Highway 5 by myself. My blond hair had suddenly turned silvery and lifeless, and my eyebrows, always healthy as caterpillars, were fading away. My skin was flaky and itchy. I was cold. My joints hurt. I had tingling in my hands and feet. My digestive system had slowed to a crawl. I couldn't sleep, and I had little appetite for anything but sushi, with a strong emphasis on tuna maki. My memory problems were still nascent, but they were gathering strength.

I figured I knew what was wrong with me. Both my mother and my sister had developed thyroid conditions at various times of their lives. I thought I might have one as well. I got the name of a local endocrinologist and made an appointment. This doctor, whose practice was geared toward the treatment of diabetes, didn't take much time with any of her patients. In fact, she booked one every ten minutes.

I sat waiting in an exam room for a long time, shivering in a blue paper sarong. When the doctor finally appeared, she stepped back and took a long look at me. Then she made a comment I don't think I'll ever forget. "Well, I agree that you look more like someone in her midfifties than a woman of forty-two," she said. What was she saying? Tears sprang into my eyes. "You're sort of weepy," she observed. "Maybe you could use some antidepressants." She ordered a blood panel, including a full complement of thyroid and reproductive hormone tests. She wrote out a prescription for Prozac, and told me to return in a couple of weeks.

When I did, she said she had good news—my tests were fine. My TSH level, thyroid-stimulating hormone, was within normal range, a perfect 3.8. She was sure the Prozac would do me good. What she didn't know was that I'd thrown it in the trash because I hated the "who gives a damn" way it made me feel. I listened to what she told me, and for the next six years, I never again considered my thyroid. Instead, I overturned every rock, looking for the source of my cognitive troubles.

Hypothyroidism has been called "the great imitator" for the vast number of medical conditions it can mimic. Thyroid imbalances may elicit fatigue, depression, coldness, constipation, poor skin, headaches, PMS, dysmenorrhea, fluid retention, weight loss or weight gain, anxiety or panic attacks, decreased memory and concentration, muscle and joint pain and low sex drive, among other symptoms. In women, who have ten times the risk of hypothyroidism that men have, the condition commonly surfaces at times when there are changes in the levels of reproductive hormones—particularly during pregnancy or menopause. The culprit is a tiny, butterfly-shaped gland at the base of the neck. When you're hypothyroid, it means that the gland isn't producing sufficient hormones to do its work—and it has an extensive job description.

In simplest terms, the thyroid is the gas pedal for every organ and cell. Thyroid hormone helps regulate virtually every cell in the body, including those in the brain. One of its most important functions is to control metabolism at the cellular level, affecting the rate at which cells use oxygen and burn energy. When you become hypothyroid, many bodily functions—including brain function—slow down. Your thyroid level affects how you use carbohydrates and protein, and how you store fat. It determines vitamin utilization, mitochondrial function, digestion, muscle and nerve activity, blood flow and oxygen utilization, hormone secretion and reproductive health.

Scientists speculate that the brain uses thyroid-stimulating hormone in the hippocampus to store and encode memory; when there is not enough TSH, or the body fails to metabolize it properly, the cognitive problems begin. One possible explanation for thyroid-related cognitive impairment is that as hypothyroidism slows the metabolism, it decreases blood flow to the hippocampus and the frontal lobes. Thyroid hormones affect the rate of cell growth in the brain, as well as the rate at which synaptic impulses travel.

Hypothyroidism results when TSH is either inadequately produced by the thyroid gland or underutilized by the blood cells. It affects an estimated thirteen million people in the United States—or maybe, many more. Among endocrinologists, who typically treat thyroid problems, there's considerable scuffling over what TSH level is normal, and what level suggests pituitary dysfunction in need of treatment. Testing labs consider TSH levels to be normal when they are between 0.4 milliunits and 4.5 milliunits—but 95 percent of Americans have TSH levels lower than 2.5, which suggests that 4.5 is far too high—and my 3.8 might be teetering on the edge. Some doctors, among them Georgetown University professor Leonard Wartoffsky, find mounting evidence that any TSH over 2.5 is abnormal and requires treatment. Lowering the TSH range would increase the percentage of the population diagnosed with hypothyroidism from 5 percent to 20 percent, an enormous leap. Many doctors think there's no need to futz around with TSH levels—that to do so will benefit no one except Abbott Laboratories, the company that manufactures Synthroid (levothyroxine), the drug most doctors prescribe when they treat hypothyroidism.

LOOK AND LISTEN

It was more or less by accident that I came upon Richard Shames. I was looking for research about hypothyroidism. He'd written some books on thyroid and hormonal disorders, and he was saying things that I thought were revolutionary. He wrote about the tyranny of TSH— how inaccurate it was, and how it precluded doctors from treating important symptoms. This time, I didn't have to travel halfway across the country to meet him. As it happened, his office was fifteen minutes up the highway.

Shames has made a science (and an art) of developing individual treatment plans for patients whose symptoms suggest thyroid imbalance, whether or not their tests reflect it. He and a growing number of thyroid specialists believe that you can't go by the tests—that the only way to accurately assess a patient is to listen and to look.

In my case, he looked and listened for over an hour. He was present and undistracted, so much so that I wondered if he was an adherent of mindfulness training. He was obviously accustomed to paying very close attention to people who had spent years trying to figure out what was wrong with them. There was nothing egotistical or grandiose about him. By the time I'd been in his office for a half hour, I realized that the endocrinologist who'd declared that my TSH was normal and I was fine didn't know her ass from her elbow. I was now in pursuit of Intervention #9.

"She had it, you know," he said, thumbing through the thick patient file I'd requested from the endocrinologist's office. "She nailed it. Thinning hair, cold hands and feet, low blood pressure, memory and concentration problems, sleep difficulties," he said, shaking his head. "And then she ignored her own diagnosis, because of the test results." That news set me on my heels. Shames began to examine me in earnest.

"Any respiratory troubles?" he asked. I told him that I had a heck of a time performing simple aerobic exercise. I could hike for miles, but put me on a treadmill, and in minutes I'd be panting like a dog.

"Air hunger"—the feeling that you simply can't get enough air into your lungs—is a common symptom of hypothyroidism. He conducted a physical exam, listening to my heart and lungs and checking my reflexes, which were anything but lively. He sent me for a long list of blood tests, far beyond the ordinary CBC. In addition to the traditional TSH, he ordered the TRH, which measures thyrotropin-releasing hormone, which, as he explained it, was like going straight to the boss, in this case the pituitary gland, which tells the thyroid what to do. Another test measured the antithyroid peroxidase (anti-TPO) antibody, which prevents the body from synthesizing thyroid hormone. In all likelihood, all tests would be in range; he suspected that my condition was one of subclinical hypothyroidism. "The tests are not gospel," he said. "With managed care and doctors trying to practice quickly and not get sued, testing has developed a preeminence it does not deserve. But it is important to actually look at the symptoms." He felt nodules in my thyroid, but these were common; he wanted to see if anything else was going on in there, so he ordered an ultrasound of the gland.

What about my memory, I asked? Sluggish brain function, he told me, is extremely common, one of the first symptoms of hypothyroidism, showing up before any other indications appeared, and patients never made the connection. Typically, he told me, there are word-retrieval problems and tip-of-the-tongue problems. "You lose your sharpness," he said. "You just don't feel as acute. This may be because not enough oxygen is getting to your brain, or because protein synthesis isn't occurring at the correct rate in the hippocampus." He left it to the scientists to figure out the exact mechanism, he said. In the meantime, he'd help people get back on track. "What I know is that it is terribly aggravating to people. I see them all the time. They come in here and tell me that they've lost their edge. Fortunately, with appropriate treatment, it's one of the first things to come back."

I told him about my experience with cognitive enhancement—that Adderall and then Provigil had worked well enough to convince me that I still had the chops. I'd just misplaced them. We agreed that we'd treat the thyroid disorder and see what happened. In the meantime, I'd leave the Provigil in the medicine cabinet.

Most practitioners, Shames said, prescribed only synthetic T-4 (Synthroid), which is converted by the liver into T-3. Some people cannot convert T-4 into T-3, no matter how much of it they have, and a common indicator of this failure is continued mental cloudiness. He suspected that I was one of the "nonconverters." After the blood tests, I would begin with a minuscule dose of T-3 (Cytomel). I would edge that dose up over the next several weeks and come back to see him. If the drug was going to help me, it would do so in that time period. We'd get results fast—before the month was up. "If you don't need Cytomel," he told me, "it's going to be too stimulating, and we'll know we have to look elsewhere." As I checked out with his receptionist, he stepped back and gave me a long look. "I have the feeling that you are not firing on all cylinders. You're a little underpowered," he said. "I think we can change that."

As Shames predicted, my TSH test was within the normal range, still hovering around 3.8. I began taking the Cytomel, in the smallest dosage available, 5 milligrams. I wasn't overstimulated—in fact, I felt very calm. As directed, after a few days I doubled the dose, to 10 milligrams. Still no jitters. Apparently, my body liked T-3.

When I next saw Richard Shames, I told him the news. I was sleeping seven hours a night, without waking up at 4:00 A.M. Seven hours might not strike some people as a great night's sleep, I told him, but for me, it was an improvement. He made note of it and asked me about my memory. There was less word loss, I told him. I wasn't in the online thesaurus every two minutes. What about my stamina? Was I able to get through more hours of work without feeling like my brain had gone on strike? Now that he mentioned it, the body pillow I kept under one of my work tables in the office and pulled out for emergency napping had gone unused for weeks.

"Okay," he said, "it's working. But looking at you, I have the sense that we have further to go." Over the next few months, he increased the Cytomel to 20 milligrams, and added a low dose of T-4, levothyroxine (Synthroid). Within days I was swimming laps easily and quickly, with no gasping for air, a problem that had plagued me for years. But all was not well: As quickly as I had found it, I lost the ability to sleep. Shames knew what had happened: "That Synthroid dose is too high for you," he said, "but it's the lowest one they make." He ordered a custom compound of levothyroxine, at about an eighth of the strength, and we had liftoff. I had tons of energy, enough to work all day, walk the dogs, and spend four happy hours in the local library with my son, teaching him how to write a research paper, I told Shames. "All good," he said with a smile. "But how's your memory?"

That was hard to say, I told him. Words came more easily, but without Provigil, my working memory continued to be impaired. That morning, flipping back and forth through an outline, I had forgotten what I was looking for in a matter of seconds. My spatial skills were, if anything, getting worse. Though I'd been there twice, I'd had to drive around the office park several times before I'd homed in on his medical building. The greatest frustration continued to be the lack of a mental grid. Where I had deposited the guest list for my son's birthday party was anybody's guess.

"With more time," Shames told me, "some of that is likely to resolve. You've got to understand that your brain has been struggling along with inadequate thyroid for many years, and function tends to return in stages." What had happened to me, he said seriously, was going to take a while to fix.

"Want to see something wild?" I asked. I pulled the clip out of my once thin and scraggly hair and let it waft to my shoulders. "It's growing like crazy," I told him. "You've got better color in your face," he observed. "You're not as pale." He tested my knee reflexes again, and leapt back as my once-lackadaisical leg shot out in his direction.

"You know," I said, "a lot of doctors think that treating subclinical thyroid disorders is inappropriate. I've also been told that too much thyroid can have a profound effect on bone metabolism—that it can cause osteoporosis."

"I'm aware of these things," he said gently. "I hope that one day, the controversy will be resolved and doctors will actually treat patients, rather than numbers." Later, he sent me a study that reviewed the effect of T-4 (Synthroid) on bone-mineral density. There is no conclusive evidence that thyroid hormone causes such troubles, but still, the possibility concerned me. "The problem," said Shames, "arises when TSH goes way out of line, into the hyperthyroid zone. You'd have to take vastly more than what you're taking now, and I'm not going to let that happen."

I believed him. For a long time, I was angry at that endocrinologist, for what seemed to me to be blatant disregard of what was written all over the patient who stood before her. If she'd treated me for subclinical hypothyroidism when I was forty-two, there was so much that I could have avoided. She was too busy to take the time to look and listen, too anxious to make her way to the patient in the exam room next door. Eventually, I realized that it wasn't entirely her fault. I'd given up too easily. I hadn't had enough confidence, or enough research behind me, to tell her I thought she was wrong. There was a lesson there for all of us, I thought: Understand that doctors are human. They are not infallible. They are often uninformed or ill-informed. They have agendas. So, do the research. Show up with the documents in hand. Make yourself crystal clear—skip that Doctor Is God routine which is ingrained in all of us. And if that doesn't work, find another doctor.

17

STARING INTO THE EYE
OF THE TIGER

. . .

Deep in the Grip of Alzheimer's Disease at the Age
of Sixty, Joanna Graciously Invites Us into Her World

As I left the freeway in my rented Chevy Malibu at Laguna Canyon Road, I understood that what lay ahead was no ordinary interview. When Joanna and I spoke on the phone, her warmth and intelligence were obvious. But her halting speech and constant search for words took their toll on us both. It would be easier, she told me, if we could meet each other in person. As I made my plans to visit, I had no idea what to expect. What would mild to moderate Alzheimer's disease look like in a fifty-nine-year-old woman? Would she even remember why I had come?

She was outside, waiting patiently for me when I finally found my way, after a series of wrong turns that made me twenty minutes late, to her cul-de-sac in Leisure World. Briefly, I considered saying something about my missing mental map, but fortunately thought better of it. Well-groomed and very fit, she wore a black-and-red knit pantsuit and matching pumps, looking for all the world like the respected family-law attorney she'd been for more than twenty years. Her white Maltese-poodle-mix puppy accompanied us up the street, past cookie-cutter 1960s vintage houses and condos. "I hate it here," Joanna said vehemently. "It's so ugly. You should have seen my beautiful house. And I hardly know anyone. The average age here is seventy-eight. I'm the youngest one by far and nobody talks to me." She sold her elegant Orange County house, with its spacious rooms and large yard, perfect for her big dog, Karlee, within weeks of her diagnosis. "I had to do it," she said. "I hadn't saved for retirement because I never expected to retire. All the money I have for the rest of my life came from that house." Within days of moving to Leisure World, Karlee got too friendly with an elderly resident, and Joanna was forced to send him to live with her grandson in North Carolina.

Although her sentences were simple, and sometimes she stalled and had to wait for me to supply a word, she was otherwise indistinguishable from any other woman her age, preparing to go out for a sociable lunch. In her small living room, she introduced me to Theo, a delightful gentleman who worked for Lockheed for forty years as a structural engineer. The two fell in love a couple of years before Joanna became ill. Through extremely difficult times, which both of them knew could only get worse, Theo had remained by her side. It was easy to see how much affection they shared. "I only wish I were not so much older than Joanna," he said when she left the room for a moment, "because it is likely that I will die long before she does, and I honestly do not know who will take care of her then."

While Joanna and I sat together on the sofa, Theo took up his place in an armchair. I hated the prospect of asking difficult questions that would cause the two of them to shed the healthy denial that allowed them to get through their days. They were cheerful, anticipating a nice lunch in a good restaurant, and I did not want to make them desperately sad.

"It's hard to explain how I knew," Joanna said. "Something was different. Something was wrong with my head. I was mad at the doctors. They . . . shoved me off. They kept saying, 'No, there's nothing wrong with you, it's hormones, it's depression,' but I knew there was more. Everything became so jumbled in my head. I couldn't keep things organized, the way I used to." Her voice trailed off. "You have to excuse me," she said. "My talking is going away now, and I'm really frustrated by that. It's the worst part. I'm not really me anymore."

Gently, Theo interrupted in his soft Greek accent, to tell Joanna that it was time to take her meds. We went together into her small, neat-as-a-pin kitchen. "She's in a drug trial," he said, "and the dosing is really complicated. You have to take a certain drug on a certain day, at a specific time, and it comes in these measured doses. It would be impossible for a person with Alzheimer's to take it without supervision." He showed me the two boxes he'd labeled for her. One was marked "Evening" and the other was marked "Morning." "There've been a few issues with the pills this week," he said matter-of-factly. "I've had to drive over several times to straighten it out." He wanted to hire a nurse's aide, but Joanna preferred his care and was reluctant to spend the money. Left unsupervised, Joanna had taken the wrong drugs at the wrong times. She'd also left the big pillbox on the kitchen table, where the puppy had gotten into it. He pointed to a list of directions, taped to the inside of the cabinet door. The first thing on the list was: Tie up the dog. It was a problem, he said, when you had so little memory. Joanna was no longer capable of doing what we do all the time—mentally retracing her steps.

Drug taking accomplished, we returned to the living room, where I surveyed a large collection of photos of her son, daughter and grandkids. Given the numbers of photos, I hoped to hear tales of a large and supportive family, but Joanna explained that neither of her children visited. I glanced at Theo. It is common for Alzheimer's patients to announce that someone never visits or calls when in fact he or she was there the previous afternoon. Theo confirmed that Joanna was right: Her children had abandoned her.

"I was the matriarch of the whole world," Joanna announced. "For so many years, I took care of everybody—the whole family. And now, nobody wants to be around me because I'm not who I was. Even my associate from the law firm, my best friend for thirty years, doesn't want to see me. I understand. She's as busy as I once was. And . . . I think maybe it's hard for people to see me like this. It hurts them. I've got too much pride to push myself on them, but I really love them and miss them."

When Joanna left the room to get fixed up for lunch, Theo confided that loneliness and depression were a big part of the problem. It was good that I came, he said. It was terrible to be afflicted at such a young age, when all of your old friends were still working and living their lives. She needed to get out much more, but who would take her? He wanted her to join a support group for people with Alzheimer's— there were plenty of them, after all, in Leisure World—but she just didn't feel any kinship with them.

We made sure that the dog was secured in the bathroom, and piled into Theo's car. On the way to lunch, Joanna told me about a trip she and Theo had taken, on a barge down a river in Burgundy. They'd danced every night on the deck. Now, when they traveled—brief domestic trips only—Theo had to put a tag on a string around her neck, on which he carefully recorded her name and the name and telephone number of their hotel. "It's still nice," Joanna said. "But it's not as nice as it used to be. I really can't keep up with him. Still, he's the most perfect man in the world." At this, Theo smiled sadly.

At King's Fish House, we settled into a crescent-shaped leather booth, with Joanna between us. She laughed a lot, especially when she failed to catch something that one of us said. She grew silent while Theo talked about what they'd been through at the hands of the physicians. Theo had been very reluctant to involve Joanna in highly experimental clinical trials, although she was exactly the kind of study participant the researchers sought. "For the average person, trying to fight this disease, it's like entering a deep, dark forest. You don't know which way to go, and any direction you choose could put you in danger," he said, patting Joanna's soft, well-manicured hand. "It's a huge responsibility. I'm a realist. I know what's coming, and that Joanna does not have much to lose. But look at her—she's young, and beautiful, and healthy in every other way. If I were to enroll her in a trial that hurt her, or made her worse, I would not be able to forgive myself. So we've ended up being very conservative in her treatment, which in retrospect was perhaps an error." I told Theo that I appreciated how difficult it must be for them—or any other Alzheimer's patient and caregiver—to remain abreast of new therapies. Every university research center had its agenda—research studies to fill with participants, papers to publish, grants to fund. There was absolutely no guarantee that a patient who presented herself as a subject for experimental therapy would end up in the trial that was best suited to her needs.

Joanna's doctor, an internist, enrolled her in an eighteen-month clinical trial of Neurochem's Alzhemed, a newer Alzheimer's drug that had shown promise in European testing. Instead of working like older drugs, which block the enzyme that degrades acetylcholine, Alzhemed interferes with the ability of beta-amyloid proteins to cling together. If they can't aggregate, they can't form plaques. When the Alzhemed trial ended, Joanna would be entitled to continue to take the drug, free of charge, for the remainder of her life.

"I think it might be working," Theo said. "I don't think I've sensed a decline during this period." Joanna also took Forest Lab's Namenda, a drug that has for years been prescribed in Germany for the treatment of moderate to severe Alzheimer's disease, but was only approved for use in the United States in late 2003. Namenda works by regulating levels of glutamate, the excitatory neurotransmitter that's integral to information processing, storage and retrieval. It may be that amyloid plaques that develop in Alzheimer's disease cause the death of glutamate receptors on nerve cells, preventing the neurotransmitter from entering the cell in sufficient amounts. Namenda increases the number of glutamate receptors, ensuring that the neurotransmitter will find an open door into the cell.

Unspoken at the table was the hope that maybe Joanna had stabilized in the mild stage of Alzheimer's. Maybe her disease would not progress to moderate and then severe stages, which are characterized by increased dependence on a caregiver, impairment in language and memory, and a drastically shortened attention span, before arriving at the profound and terminal stages that precede death. Only time would tell.

Theo and I were unbearably full of fish, spinach and potatoes, but Joanna ordered a big dish of vanilla ice cream for dessert. It was so good, she said enthusiastically, that I had to taste it. I grabbed my spoon and dug in, feeling like part of the family.

Theo asked me to tell them what I knew about the most promising research in the field. Was there a new clinical trial they ought to consider for Joanna, when the Alzhemed study ended, especially if things began to get worse?

CLINICAL TRIALS

As I discussed earlier, scientists believe that an accumulation of still-soluble proteins may represent the earliest evidence of Alzheimer's disease. These proteins are capable of blocking communications between cells, resulting in the mild forgetfulness we associate with middle age. For some people, that's as far as it goes, but for others, these tiny proteins trigger a series of steps, called the amyloid cascade, which lead to the development of beta-amyloid plaques and neurofibrillary tangles, thick, sticky gobs of cellular proteins that strangle nerve cells. It's an ongoing molecular process involving a slow accumulation of cellular garbage—misfolded proteins, unhinged amino acids—that the neuronal housekeeper has failed to sweep away.

The first generation of Alzheimer's drugs, the acetylcholinesterase inhibitors, Aricept and Donepezil among them, break down the enzyme that destroys the neurotransmitter acetylcholine, temporarily increasing communication between failing neurons.

The real target for intervention is much further upstream—very possibly in the soluble proteins that begin to accumulate in midlife. There are drugs in the pipeline that could prevent these proteins from aggregating, and even help to clear them after they've begun to cling to each other, long before nerve cells start to die.

There were at least half a dozen human clinical trials in progress that were worth considering, I told Theo and Joanna. Some were small Phase 1 and Phase 2 studies, where safety is the main focus. Others had made it into Phase 3, where drugs and therapies were tested to see whether what has worked in mice will also be effective in people. These trials weren't for everybody. Things could go wrong. Rarely, they went so wrong that people perished. But if they wanted my opinion, I believed it was worth the risk in order to treat the disease as aggressively as possible. One did not have to lie down in the path of this bulldozer.

There was, for example, the COGNIshunt study, which began at the University of Pennsylvania and continues, with promising results, at Stanford. A tiny valve, intended to filter undesirable substances from the bloodstream, was placed under the skin at the base of the skull. More tubing extended from there to the peritoneum, a space in the belly where fluids accumulate before flowing into the kidneys to be filtered and eliminated in the urine. The shunt, which has the selective capacity to filter out toxins of a specific molecular weight and size, reduces the levels of isoprostanes and misfolded proteins by about 50 percent. The MMSE scores of patients who were treated with the shunt remained stable, while the scores of those who did not receive it declined by about 20 percent.

Over the years, researchers have observed that during the early stages of Alzheimer's disease, insulin levels and insulin receptors decline dramatically. Insulin and a related protein, IGF-1, appear to be responsible for stimulating the expression of the enzyme that makes acetylcholine, which you may recall also drops precipitously in the initial stages of the disease. By the time a patient is in the terminal stage of Alzheimer's, insulin levels are nearly 80 percent lower than they are in a normal brain. Suzanne Craft, the scientist who studies the relationship between insulin, acetylcholine levels and Alzheimer's, is developing treatments that use nose drops to deliver insulin directly to the brain. Volunteers who received intranasal insulin experienced memory improvement in three different neuropsychological tests. Follow-up studies will examine whether daily administration of insulin spray may be helpful to people with memory problems.

Another approach to treating Alzheimer's disease enlists the body's immune system to clean up the plaques and tangles. At university research centers in more than eighteen states, Elan Pharmaceuticals is currently testing bapineuzumab, a monoclonal antibody (also referred to as AAB-001) that binds to and clears beta-amyloid protein in its nascent stage. The new vaccine shows promise at clearing both soluble and deposited forms of amyloid in mice and in humans who have come to autopsy after the completion of their trial. At the University of California, Irvine, Frank LaFerla is testing AF267B, a disease-modifying compound that works by boosting the level of an enzyme called alpha secretase, which prevents the production of beta-amyloid. The drug also enhances the activity of receptors for acetylcholine. Results so far are promising: The drug seems to reduce the severity of plaques and tangles in the hippocampus, which may make it the first compound that can reverse damage that has already occurred.

Scientists at New York Presbyterian Hospital/Weill Cornell Medical Center are currently running a trial of intravenous immuglobulin therapy, called IVIg, which has already proved to be successful in treating immune diseases and hepatitis. It involves an infusion of antibodies derived from human plasma that latch on to abnormal proteins and clear them from the nervous system. In the preliminary phase of the trial, eight Alzheimer's patients were treated with IVIg for six months, and then tested for cognitive function, which improved in six study participants and remained stable for one. Tests of cerebrospinal fluid in each of the participants on average showed a 45 percent decrease in the level of beta-amyloid. Those numbers, I told Joanna, were quite impressive, particularly since IVIg has already passed the FDA's safety requirements for the treatment of other diseases, and thus would not be as risky as some of the other therapies.

In the past year, much closer to home, there was another investigation, perhaps the boldest of them all, involving gene therapy. Since 1987, scientists at the University of California, San Diego have been perfecting a gene therapy technique that allows them to insert extra copies of a gene, riding on the back of a gene therapy virus, into the brains of Alzheimer's patients. Subjects receive the implanted grafts into targeted areas through two holes drilled on either side of the skull. Once in place, the virus switches on the gene that expresses nerve growth factor (NGF), a naturally occurring protein that prevents cell death and stimulates the function of acetylcholine-producing neurons. PET scans of NGF gene therapy show that neurons regain function. Intriguingly, mental status tests showed a reduction in cognitive decline of 36 to 51 percent. The best test scores were submitted more than six months after surgery, which means that it took several months for the cells to receive the full benefit of the elevated level of nerve growth factor. When investigators examined the brain tissue of a participant who died of other causes, they found robust growth emerging from cells that produce acetylcholine, the same cells that are the first to degenerate in the very early stages of Alzheimer's. In recent months, the investigation has been transferred from the UCSD laboratory of Mark Tuszynski—who developed the procedure—to Georgetown University, where the Phase 2 open-enrollment randomized clinical trial is underway. In this investigation, one group of patients received extra copies of the nerve growth factor gene, while the control group was subjected to sham surgery in which a scalp incision was made, but no needle was passed into the brain. Over the next year, the study will expand to other clinical settings. They've had good results, but the surgery has its limitations, warns Tuszynski. Because neurons that produce acetylcholine must still be alive to benefit from the elevated nerve growth factor, the surgery is effective only in the early stages of Alzheimer's disease. Nor will this gene therapy cure the disease. "It slows down decline for several years," says Tuszynski, "and that's worth a lot. But eventually, amyloid proteins will encroach upon other types of neurons, and kill them."

"That sounds good," Joanna said to Theo after I finished describing the implant process, as if she was talking about something short-term like a weekend in Los Angeles. "Should we try for that?"

"Would you really do it?" I asked, remembering what Theo had said about keeping her treatment as conservative as possible. "Would you try something that screwed around with your genes?"

"Definitely, I would," she said. "I think it's really important for me to be out there, volunteering for things. I really want to keep living. There's going to be a cure, and if I can be the first one who gets it, that's good, isn't it?"

When I told Theo that I would forward him all the information I could find about new trials and promising developments, I saw Joanna register my assumption that she wouldn't be able to understand. Instantly, I was sorry. I tried to imagine how it felt to suffer such put-downs—however inadvertent—every single day.

"I'm a determined person," she said. "I'm so healthy. I've never been healthier in my life. It's just that I'm losing my mind. But I don't give up. I never do."

After lunch, Joanna shared with me what she had not shared with anybody besides Theo. Since early childhood, her hippocampus had been besieged. As a young girl, she'd suffered sexual abuse at the hands of her stepfather. She spent the remainder of her childhood, well into her twenties, caring for her alcoholic mother and raising her two younger siblings. She'd suffered from post-traumatic stress disorder and clinical depression throughout her life. I asked if her doctors had ever mentioned that PTSD and depression increased the risk of developing Alzheimer's disease. She said they had not.

Theo spun us back to Joanna's place. It was time for her to take a rest. They had a big night ahead: They were off to a concert of classical music at South Coast Symphony. As we approached the cul-de-sac, Theo asked me where I had parked my rental car. Although I'd made careful note of the model and the color, I realized that I had no idea what it looked like, or for that matter, why it was not parked out in front of Joanna's house. As if in a video, I had to rewind, zipping backward through the neurofootage until I reached the place where Joanna was standing outside with the puppy, directing me into a visitor's space a block from her residence. What if I couldn't do that? What if that rewind function simply wasn't available to me? That was Joanna's life now, and it would get worse.

As I prepared for what I knew would be a very long rush-hour drive to Los Angeles, Theo issued directions. "Now, to leave here, you'll take a left, and then another left, and then a right, at which point you'll come to the guard gate, and when you pass through, you'll take a left. When you see the shopping center where we ate lunch, bear to the right, and then you'll see the freeway, where you'll head north." His instructions were crystal clear, but he might as well have been speaking in his native Greek. By the time I stepped on the accelerator, they had left my brain forever.

THE DISEASE TAKES OVER

I stayed in close touch with Theo over the course of a year. I sent him information about the LaFerla study in San Diego, and the gene therapy study. Joanna was still enrolled in the Alzhemed trial, which precluded her from joining most other medication trials, and to Theo, the gene therapy study seemed too drastic an approach. But time was slipping away. At sixty, Joanna's condition was declining visibly, he wrote in an e-mail. Her ability to communicate and follow simple instructions had diminished markedly. He warned me that she was quickly being subsumed by the disease. She required constant caretaking—most recently, she had forgotten how to use the key she wore on a ribbon around her neck, which left her standing for a very long time outside her own front door. That marked the end of her freedom.

I wanted to see her again, so I arranged with Theo to visit on a Sunday afternoon, after he picked Joanna up from church, one of the few places she could still go alone. I recalled how much she'd enjoyed our lunch at the fish restaurant, so I suggested that we head down to Laguna Beach to have some cool drinks on the broad terrace overlooking the sea at the Montage Resort. Then we'd go out to dinner, my treat.

Joanna and Theo were waiting at the curb when I got off the train. Theo gave me his usual gracious greeting, insisting on managing my overnight bag and my briefcase, but I could see the pain in his face. Joanna looked terrific. She'd lost a little weight, and had a spiky new haircut that suited her. As she smiled benignly, I realized that she was regarding me as one might a total stranger, although I knew that Theo had reminded her many times that I was coming. After a few minutes of talking about our last visit—the fish lunch, the vanilla ice cream—she seemed to know who I was. But easy conversation, such as we had before, was impossible. So many words were missing that she could barely construct a short sentence.

"I want my car," she said angrily. "I miss my car." Theo had already filled me in: She could no longer drive—she'd gotten lost for five hours, on her way home from the market, and had to be retrieved by the police. "And there are people coming in and out of my house, all the time, rifling through my things," she said.

I looked to Theo for guidance on this one. He had mentioned that the delusions were increasing in frequency.

"Are there, dearest?" he asked brightly. "How do they get in?"

"Through the door, of course," she said, brimming with irritation. "They all have keys. They take my glasses and my makeup and toss everything around so I can't find . . . anything." I noticed that she was crying, and passed a box of tissues from the backseat to the front.

Even before we arrived at the Montage, I knew it was a mistake. The parking area was crowded with fancy cars and showy people, and Joanna, in her practical blue jeans and T-shirt, clutched my hand tightly as we walked through the lobby. Remarkably, we got a table right away. When I invited her to join me on a trip to the ladies' room, Theo looked relieved. At least he wouldn't have to deal with that. She held my hand all the way there, and I found myself checking—as I used to do when my children were toddlers—that she hadn't left the restroom while I was still in the stall.

Back at the table, we talked of our favorite places. Theo loved his native Greece, and he and Joanna were planning to take a final trip there this summer. I must have raised a skeptical eyebrow.

"I will be eighty next fall," he said simply. "I'm not leaving her home, so she will come with me. Somehow, we will manage."

Joanna talked about Mount Shasta, in northern California, recalling many fishing trips to an area I'd also visited, called Castle Crags Wilderness. She used to hop in the car with her kids, she said, and drive the whole ten hours herself.

"I'd love to see that again," she said wistfully. "If I had my car, I could go."

Theo and I exchanged glances. Was it possible? Could we take her there? If we did, would she recall that she wanted to go, and that she'd been there before, or would she just be terrified?

"Maybe Theo and I could take you there," I ventured, afraid of promising something that would be impossible to deliver.

"I'd do all the driving," she volunteered. "I love to drive. You know, they've taken my car away and I want to have it back."

As the afternoon wore into evening, Joanna grew tired. Her words deserted her, and her anger flared. There was more discussion about the people who slipped into her house—young women, mostly—and took her things. I suggested that it might be a great idea to have the locks changed; surely, that would take care of the problem. Joanna shook her head sadly and told me that it wouldn't help—these people would find new keys, or, as she'd observed occasionally, they'd slip through the walls.

I could tell that Theo was running on empty. This was not how he'd intended to finish out his years. And yet, he stayed. There were still a couple of hours left until my flight, but he and Joanna took me to the Orange County airport, that palace of marble and gilt, more akin to a luxury shopping mall than a transportation hub. There, I threw myself down in a leather seat, shaken and exhausted. In a year, despite the trial of Alzhemed and the prescription for Namenda, the disease had wrought unspeakable havoc. In the time I had known Joanna, she had passed from mild Alzheimer's to a much more advanced stage of pathology. By the next time I saw her, I suspected that she would not know me, and no amount of reminiscing would restore her memory.

18

DO YOU REALLY WANT TO KNOW?

. . .

As Opportunities for Early Assessment
and Intervention Become Available,
Will You Embrace Them?

As awareness of Alzheimer's disease increases, and opportunities for early intervention surface, it is likely that more middle-aged people will demand to be evaluated. "I'd welcome knowing about Alzheimer's at the earliest possible moment," wrote Rudy, an audio-equipment manufacturer, "so that I could document the essence of myself for my son and younger friends, before it was too late."

Some concerned individuals will find their way to excellent university research centers, but most will discuss their problems with their primary care physicians, who may well be uninformed or misinformed about newer approaches to diagnosing and treating the disease. One internist, whose suburban patients are mostly high-income professionals deeply concerned about maintaining their cognitive skills, told me that nearly every one of his middle-aged patients mentioned that his or her memory was slipping. Inaccurately, he explained to me that it is easy to distinguish Alzheimer's symptoms from "normal" age-related memory impairment. "If a person is worried about his memory, that tells me his problem is stress or depression," he said. "People with Alzheimer's disease don't know there's anything wrong. They're convinced they're just fine."

"That's so typical," said Ron Peterson, who directs the neurology department at the Mayo Alzheimer's Disease Center in Rochester, Minnesota. "You finally work up the nerve to go in and talk to your physician. You say, 'Hey, I've been having some trouble with words and people's names' and the physician says, 'Guess what, so have I, join the club.' We're trying to raise awareness among physicians so these concerns will not be brushed off."

Thinking about Joanna, Stuart, Ralph, and Bruce, all of whom spent months in the hands of primary care physicians who assured them that they'd just been working too hard, I wanted to smack that internist for his cluelessness. He'd never learned that the seeds of Alzheimer's disease were planted in middle age, or that a patient who complained of a decline in cognition ought to be taken seriously.

But how were primary care physicians to sort through the dozens of patients who were concerned about forgetfulness, in order to find the few who really needed help? Surely, it was not feasible to send these otherwise healthy midlife patients off for neuropsych tests, MRIs and PET scans, which are expensive and subject to misinterpretation.

LOOKING FOR BIOMARKERS

John Q. Trojanowski, the director of the Penn Institute on Aging and Alzheimer's Disease at the University of Pennsylvania, is well aware of the conundrum. "We need more diagnostic accuracy," he said, "an approach that's much more specific. It's got to be simple, inexpensive and accurate—the equivalent of a pregnancy test." That's his goal, as an investigator in the Alzheimer's Disease Neuroimaging Initiative, a $60 million, five-year study at fifty sites across the United States and Canada involving eight hundred people aged fifty-five to ninety. Funded by the National Institute on Aging, The National Institutes of Health and a half-dozen major pharmaceutical companies, the initiative aims to find a foolproof method of diagnosing Alzheimer's disease at the earliest possible stage. "If we can find that, in a safe, noninvasive form," said Trojanowski, "patients will insist on having it."

Trojanowski heads the Neuroimaging Initiative's hunt for Alzheimer's biomarkers, which measure the level of a particular substance in the blood, urine, plasma or cerebrospinal fluid. Such markers exist at various levels of sophistication for many diseases—there's hemoglobin A1c for diabetes, and cholesterol and CRP test for heart disease.

"What we're doing," Trojanowski explained, "is looking for diagnostic laboratory tests that will distinguish Alzheimer's disease from other neurological degeneration that can look a lot like it." Alzheimer's can be confused with vascular dementia, Parkinsonian dementia, frontotemporal dementia, dementia with Lewy bodies, Pick's disease and primary progressive aphasia. "We need a test that is age-blind," he continued, "meaning that you can give it to a forty-year-old or an eighty-year-old, without having the results confounded by age-related factors." A single biomarker, he added, was unlikely to do the job. A panel of markers, including a biomarker, a hippocampal scan and a neuropsychological test of delayed recall, could pinpoint trouble before it emerged fullblown.

He and his colleagues have already found a few promising biomarkers, measuring levels of isoprostane, tau, beta-amyloid, sulfatide and homocysteine. So far, the most promising markers exist in cerebrospinal fluid, which flows through the extracellular spaces in the brain. In CSF, it is already possible to track some biomarkers with high sensitivity. But because these biomarkers appear only in CSF, obtained through an invasive and painful procedure known as a spinal tap, they're not ready for prime time. Trojanowski is extremely optimistic. "Within months, or at most a couple of years, we'll find what we need, and early assessment will be a reality. That's very important, because pharmaceutical companies are paving the way for early intervention with next-generation anti-amyloid drugs."

NEW APPROACHES TO SCANNING

The hippocampal scan to which Trojanowski refers is the brainchild of a research team at New York University, led by Mony de Leon, M.D. He and his colleagues have developed an image-analysis technique that quickly and accurately measures volume and metabolic activity in the hippocampus, compares it to the norm and spits out an answer. The program allows researchers to standardize and automate the sampling of PET brain scans. "Right now," notes de Leon, "we can show with great accuracy who will develop Alzheimer's disease nine years in advance of symptoms, and our projections suggest we might be able to take that out as far as fifteen years. This is push-button stuff. It's not just about getting the image—anyone who can operate a scanner can do that. This is about getting the fully interpreted results." De Leon's goal is to collect enough information to be able to set standards that would allow doctors to pinpoint the earliest stages of the disease, even in otherwise healthy young people.

Where does that leave Gary Small's PET scans? "I don't think they're ready to stand on their own," John Trojanowski told me. "Gary will say, 'No, we're there,' but I think that my peers and colleagues who work in this field know that this is wishful thinking. We're clearly not there yet."

Hearing that—and similar comments from several esteemed researchers in the field—I wondered if the PET scan I'd undergone at UCLA was actually predictive of anything or if I'd juiced myself with radioactive isotope to no avail. After a long interview in his offices at New York University Hospital, I asked Mony de Leon if he would review my scans and let me know what he thought about my hippocampus. Most graciously, he agreed. Upon my return to California, I mailed him the three-foot-long brown envelope containing my films. A few weeks went by, and then he called.

"It's nothing but good news," he said. "It's a great-looking hippocampus. In fact, it's quite a normal-looking brain. To be honest, I don't even see the wear and tear on it that you might expect to see in a person younger than you are. Your MRI shows that it is normal, robustly normal—and believe me, MRI is so sensitive that if you wake up on the wrong side of the bed, you're going to see it." For a moment I felt as if someone had just underestimated my age by a decade. "When we have verifiable memory problems—like your bad scores on your neuropsych exam—at least 70 percent of the time, we see a problem on the scan. The fact that your hippocampus looks so perfect would lead me to believe that whatever problems you are experiencing come from some other source."

Another group at NYU is developing a method of assessment that looks very promising, using electroencephalogram technology. I smiled when I read the article in *Neurobiology and Aging*: Good old Marvin Sams, the electrophysiologist who'd conducted my neurofeedback training, would surely get a kick out of knowing that the relatively unsophisticated machines and electrodes he swore by were now in the news, predicting with 90 percent accuracy in healthy people in their sixties and seventies who would develop Alzheimer's within seven years, and with 95 percent accuracy whose cognitive abilities would remain virtually unchanged. The procedure took thirty minutes to perform, required no injections or tedious stints in banging MRI machines. The most important finding? Subjective complaints— a subject's feeling that his memory was faltering—turned out to be a significant predictor of decline. "The abnormalities we detected were not subtle at all," said lead investigator Leslie S. Prichep. "They were so deviant from normal aging values that there's no doubt in my mind that when we look back even earlier, we'll still pick up abnormalities."

A GENETIC MARKER

Although it remains highly controversial, there's at least one additional predictor of who will develop Alzheimer's disease. The apolipoprotein gene, known as ApoE, resides on chromosome 19. Everybody carries two copies of it, one from each parent. The ApoE gene, like all others, is subject to polymorphisms, or slight variants, which scientists refer to as alleles. In this particular gene, the alleles are called E2, E3 and E4. People who carry a single E4 variant—between 20 and 30 percent of the population—have three to five times the risk of developing Alzheimer's disease as those who carry the E2 or the E3 variant. People who carry two copies of the E4 allele have about fifteen times the risk of developing the disease as noncarriers. On average, E4 carriers show symptoms of memory decline seven years earlier than those with E2 or E3 alleles.

You'd expect such a genetic marker to be a valuable predictor of who will develop the disease. But there's a hitch: ApoE is a susceptibility gene, rather than a deterministic one, which is to say that it raises the probability that you will develop Alzheimer's, but by no means ensures it. Some people who carry double E4 alleles never become ill, while one-third of people who do develop Alzheimer's do not carry the E4 variant. In short, as a predictor, ApoE is far from perfect.

ApoE is a protein that helps shuttle cholesterol and other nonsoluble lipid particles around the body, moving these substances to where they are needed, to provide quick energy, to store as fat for later use or to repair wounds. In the brain, ApoE functions as a street sweeper. It picks up lipids and other materials that result from brain wear and tear, or from trauma, and transports them to where they can be used or cleared. Recent studies suggest that, compared to the lively behavior of the E2 and E3 alleles, E4 is a laggard, allowing protein aggregates and other debris to accumulate.

The E4 allele is currently being held responsible for all sorts of cellular havoc. It increases the risk of diabetes, raises total cholesterol and makes smoking far more dangerous. People who carry E4 and drink alcohol are four times more likely to develop dementia than people who do not drink. Although supplementary estrogen notably improves learning and memory in women who carry the E2 and E3 allele, it appears to have no effect on women who carry E4. Individuals who carry the E4 variant also show more depressive symptomatology, as well as reduced evidence of the birth of new cells and the healthy proliferation of dendrites in the hippocampus. Myelin, the fatty coating that protects axons, breaks down faster in the presence of E4, slowing communication between neurons.

The mutant protein may also interfere with neurons' ability to make use of glucose. In PET imaging of cognitively normal subjects—in their teens and twenties, as well as in midlife—people who carried the E4 variant consistently demonstrated reduced glucose metabolism in the same regions of the brain as those who had already been diagnosed with probable Alzheimer's disease. People who carry the E4 variant also show more frontal-lobe functional impairment when they are under stress: Put too much pressure on them, and they can't think straight.

Given the broad implications of this list, I found it hard to imagine why doctors weren't ordering this straightforward blood test for practically everyone. Surely it would be useful to be able to say to a patient, "Hey, pal, you just came up with a couple of E4s, so if you think you're doing yourself a favor with the red wine at dinner, think again."

ApoE genotyping seemed so logical and practical I was shocked to learn that very few scientists or physicians believed that ordering this test was a good idea. Even Allen Roses, the Duke University scientist who found the E4 alelle in 1995, advised physicians against ordering the test except as a method of confirming Alzheimer's pathology in patients who already have a diagnosis of unspecified progressive dementia. In fact, federal regulations prohibit ordinary people from learning their ApoE genotype. The information is not disclosed out of fear that it will be misunderstood and produce adverse psychological consequences. Several expert consensus conferences have concluded that the risk of misunderstanding outweighs the potential benefits.

Slowly, as scientists get closer to producing viable therapies for

Alzheimer's, researchers are beginning to question this paternalistic stance. At the forefront of that movement is Robert Green, a professor of neurology, genetics and epidemiology, as well as the associate director of the Alzheimer's Disease Center at Boston University's School of Public Health. Green divides his time between caring for Alzheimer's patients and their families in a clinical setting and running what is arguably one of the most controversial research programs in the country. I met him at his office, and liked him immediately. In contraposition to the scholarly argyle-knit vest he wore over a crisply starched dress shirt, his chin sported a very funky and youthful soulpatch.

As the principal investigator and director of REVEAL, which is funded by the Human Genome Project, Green and his team disclose the ApoE genotype to study participants. "We have all sorts of safety checks and balances in place," he told me, "including licensed genetic counselors who dispense information." Participants receive careful psychological monitoring before they have the blood test and after they get the results.

"It is certainly true," Green explained, "that your ApoE genotype does not determine whether or not you are going to get Alzheimer's. But having that information on hand can help us select individuals who are at high risk, so when treatments that might delay or prevent the development of Alzheimer's become available, we know who to target. ApoE is the most powerful presymptomatic risk factor ever discovered for Alzheimer's disease, and it's evident that it's a huge risk factor for conversion from mild memory problems to full-blown pathology."

In the process of setting up the protocol for REVEAL, a study that has now been underway for six years, Green's team contacted a large database of individuals, mostly middle-aged or older, who had first-degree relatives with Alzheimer's. More than 20 percent of those who were contacted proceeded through the blood-draw step, a total of five hundred people in two phases of the study. "Here we have a genetic test that's not a very precise measure of disease risk," noted Green, "for a disorder for which there is still no cure, and yet 23 percent of a systematically contacted population was prepared to come in, sign up, go through the counseling, and have their blood drawn. To me, this is a remarkable finding. It means that there are potentially millions of people out there who want to know."

I mentioned my conversation with Robert Green to one of the survey participants, a Boston woman in her late forties whose mother was in late-stage Alzheimer's. Her maternal aunt had already died in the grip of the disease, and another, younger aunt was starting to show symptoms of decline. Caroline was in a panic. During the course of her mother's long illness, she'd learned nothing about early diagnosis, innovations in treatment, or what she, herself, might do to stave off this fate. When she shared her concerns with her own doctor, "He was weirdly dismissive," she said, "as if it was something that did not bear talking about." I told Caroline that Robert Green's REVEAL study might help her define her level of risk, and she asked for a phone number.

"That's not unusual at all," said Green when I told him I'd like to refer Caroline to the study. "When a daughter comes in with the parent, she is not the identified patient. By the time the mother goes downhill and is put in a nursing home, the daughter doesn't even see the doctor anymore. The doctors never see the iceberg of fear in the adult child, and the adult children don't speak of it because it seems selfish and neurotic."

Several months later, I phoned Caroline to see if she'd enrolled in REVEAL. She'd been to the lab, where they'd done the blood test, a neuropsych test and another to measure anxiety and depression. Within a couple of weeks, she'd received word that her results were ready. She returned to the lab, and a researcher showed her a graph of her statistical likelihood of developing Alzheimer's. "It was 52 percent," Caroline said. "Frankly, I'd assumed that my risk was a great deal higher—that it was more or less inevitable that I'd get it, too. For the first time in a long while, I had a feeling that there was hope. It wasn't a done deal that I would die in the same way as my relatives. To some extent, I went through this to kick myself out of denial, and it worked. It forced me to get out there and take better care of myself, to lose weight, to keep my stress level down, to have social interaction—everything I'm supposed to do to keep my brain in trim. It was very motivating."

I asked Robert Green if he could arrange for me to have the ApoE test. I'd just found a new study showing that E4 carriers who'd experienced head trauma had a significantly higher risk of developing Alzheimer's disease than people who carried the E2 and E3 alleles. After inquiring about my genetic history—three grandparents who died before they were sixty-five (from stroke, heart failure and suicide), one who remained remarkably intact into her early nineties, and two parents who were in robust health—he told me that without a first-degree relative who died of Alzheimer's disease, he could not enroll me in REVEAL. It was unlikely, he said, that I would be able to get the test on my own. I'd need a diagnosis of unspecified dementia, which for several reasons—my continued possession of a driver's license and my ability to secure health insurance among them—I did not want.

My internist, who at this point was accustomed to requests from me for odd laboratory tests, simply noted "memory impairment" in the appropriate column on the laboratory form and faxed the order to Quest, the local blood lab. From there, it traveled to Athena Diagnostics, a laboratory in Worcester, Massachusetts, that in 1995 licensed the exclusive worldwide patent rights to diagnostic uses of Duke University's ApoE4 test. Over several weeks, I received calls and letters from Athena, any of which would have flummoxed a patient suffering from dementia. They required additional insurance information. They needed a different code from my doctor. They wished to discuss insurance coverage—would I be willing to pay a $90 flat fee as part of their patient advocate program? I paid up, and they assured me that the results were in the mail. A week later, when the paperwork failed to arrive, I called Athena again. Introducing myself this time as a member of the press, I asked some pointed questions of a media contact who had apparently been deputized in order to deflect my inquiries. Repeatedly, she recommended that I visit the Web site, where it specifically stated that what I was trying to do was impossible. I assumed I'd lost the battle, but a week after my discussion with the media contact, my doctor's receptionist called to say that the results had come in. I carried no E4 alleles—I was an E2 and E3 gal. I could drink that small glass of red wine with dinner without concern for anything other than the headache I'd have in the morning. The various blows I'd taken to the head didn't put me at any higher risk for developing Alzheimer's than anyone else. I wondered if I'd have felt different if two E4 alleles had popped up. Would I have lost heart and momentum?

For the two lively ApoE variants, I was grateful. I also relished the clean bill of health Mony de Leon had produced for my hippocampus. I suspected that I'd already begun to retrieve some of the cognitive ability I thought was lost forever. Now all I had to do was to make sure that my brain remained in the best possible shape for the decades to come.

19

EMERGING TRIUMPHANT

. . .

How to Stockpile Neurons:

The Habits of the Cognitively Well-Endowed

What, besides motherly concern, allowed Eleanor of Aquitaine, at seventy-eight, to lead an army into battle to crush a rebellion against the reign of her son, King James? Why, at the advanced age of eighty-six, was choreographer Martha Graham able to raise the curtain on her newest work, *Maple Leaf Rag*? What kept George Bernard Shaw writing lucidly into his nineties and permitted Oliver Wendell Holmes to preside over the Supreme Court until he retired at ninety-one? Which exceptional segments of DNA allowed Alan Greenspan to remain chairman of the Federal Reserve for eighteen years, until he stepped down at age seventy-nine? It's unlikely (with the possible exception of Greenspan) that any of these people swallowed daily doses of coenzyme Q-10 or alpha-lipoic acid.

Why do some people's brains remain extremely sharp into old age?

It's possible: Five percent of people between the ages of e
eighty-nine score as well on tests of verbal recall as the
teen-year-old. Nobel Prize winner Eric Kandel, seventy-six, w.....
regarded as the father of learning and memory research, laid out the
explanation for me in his spacious office at Columbia University. A
lean, bow-tied gentleman whose gracious manner reflects his Austrian
roots, he beamed at me from behind saucer-size tortoiseshell spec-
tacles. Wisps of wild white hair flew from above his impressively large
ears. Kandel's laboratory has been instrumental in revealing much of
what we know about brain plasticity. Memory Pharmaceuticals, the
company he started in 1998 and where he serves as chief scientific officer, is at the forefront of the race to develop drugs that may counteract
age-associated memory impairment, and its more severe relative, mild
cognitive impairment.

"There soon may be a little red pill you take every day, something
like an aspirin," he said. "But it would be a gross error to rely on this
in middle age, or any time. Genetics play a part in this. But what you
do with your mind all through your life will to a large degree determine the course of your old age.

"If you were to ask me how you might assure that your intellectual functions continue unperturbed into your eighties or nineties, I
would say that you should continue to work," he observed. "In fact,
you should take on difficult tasks in areas that are new to you. Learn
another language, study an area of mathematics or engineering or art."
In addition to the challenges he faces each day at Columbia, running
a scientific entity so famous that it is known only as "the Kandel lab,"
and charting the course of Memory Pharmaceuticals, he swims several
times a week, and stretches and lifts light weights almost daily to keep
himself in shape for the tennis he plays on the weekends. He and his
wife visit museums and galleries about once a week, in the interest of
enhancing their collection of Austrian and German expressionist art
and art nouveau furniture and vases. They also have a subscription to
the Metropolitan Opera. "I don't do anything very unusual," he tells
me, but I get the picture: If you're not climbing, you're probably slipping.

STOCKPILING NEURONS

Down the block and around the corner at the Taub Institute, there's another Columbia scientist, neuropsychologist Yaakov Stern, who has pledged much of his career to revealing the underpinnings of the "climbing-slipping" hypothesis. He studies how people develop "cognitive reserve," which he describes as a sort of neuronal padding, added over a lifetime. His research has shown that although childhood IQ and educational and occupational opportunities play significant roles in determining cognitive reserve, leisure activities are also important.

Stern's studies suggest that individuals who are equipped with better-than-average levels of cognitive reserve maintain high levels of function despite the progressive neuronal degeneration that comes with normal aging. Noting that rodents exposed to greater physical and mental stimulation show increased levels of neurogenesis, as well as denser dendritic branching and a substantial increase in the number of synaptic connections, he theorized that the same events occur in humans, although there is no direct way to measure neural density and connectivity. "It appears," he said, "that individuals who are equipped with high levels of reserve have a more flexible brain software. They don't dead-end as easily when faced with a complex cognitive challenge, perhaps because they're accustomed to considering multiple approaches. They are able to switch networks, to transfer operations rapidly from the temporal lobes to the frontal lobes, if the temporal lobes can no longer do the job efficiently. It's all about the brain's ability to switch to plan B. What gives people with high reserve the upper hand is the ability to summon the compensatory response." Neuropsychologist Elkhonon Goldberg, author of *The Executive Brain*, a book about frontal-lobe function, observes that "a greater functional longevity of the frontal lobes is an important key to a sound mind in advanced age. Those who preserve a good working condition of their frontal lobes are the ones with the best chance of remaining clear-minded into old age." Goldberg notes that people with lifelong histories of complex executive decision making tend to perform better in old age "than passive 'follower types' with relatively modest exertion of their executive function."

In youth, when faced with a challenging memory task, your hippocampus, deep in the temporal lobe, settled down to work, occasionally calling in the right hemisphere of your frontal lobe. With age, as hippocampal function declines, and the right frontal lobe is on duty all the time, the left frontal lobe must also be recruited. People who are able to achieve bilateral activation are often especially insightful—what some call wise. They have access to the extensive library of patterns they've stored over the years. Two-sided activation allows them to see things, quite readily, that people with less integrated brains cannot. Still, there's a downside to bilateral activation you may be aware of at this moment. On certain tasks, involving concentration and multitasking, it's as if the two hemispheres are jostling with each other to be first in line. Not surprisingly, you wind up scatterbrained.

Stern and his colleagues studied the autopsied brains of individuals with Alzheimer's, whose cognitive states had been carefully tracked for years before they died. "What we found," he said, "was that when we compared the brains of two people who clinically were in the same stage of the disease at the time of death, the person with higher cognitive reserve showed a greater accumulation of the plaques and tangles that are part of the pathology of Alzheimer's." This suggested that the high-reserve person had been able to "hide" the debilitating symptoms of the disease, possibly for years.

I have to admit that this hypothesis puzzled me until I encountered a startling example in the excellent British science magazine, *New Scientist*. The article described the case of Robert Wetherill, a retired university lecturer who "was intolerably good at chess . . . able to think a mind-boggling eight moves ahead." The professor was dismayed, reporter Lisa Melton explained, when his razor-sharp mind started to dull, and he could only think five moves ahead. He was certain that something was seriously wrong, and sought out the help of neurologist Nick Fox at University College's London Institute of Neurology. Fox's battery of tests revealed nothing amiss; according to Melton, the "patient sailed through every test designed to spot early dementia." Two years later, in 2003, when Wetherill suddenly died, Fox performed an autopsy and discovered a brain chock-full of plaques and tangles. "The anatomical evidence indicated advanced disease," wrote Melton, "with a level of physical damage that would have reduced most people to a state of confusion." Yet for Wetherill—who had developed a high level of cognitive reserve—the only impact was that he could no longer play chess to high standards. The professor's intellectually stimulating life had apparently allowed him to carry on as usual and remain lucid up to the moment of his death, despite the high levels of accumulating toxins in his brain.

Compared to individuals with lower levels of education and IQ, those with a high level of cognitive reserve have a 46 percent reduced risk of developing dementia. "The idea," said Stern, "is that a high cognitive reserve might keep you from developing the disease for enough years so that you die of something else."

It's worth noting a sad irony. Very high-functioning individuals like Wetherill invariably ace the simple neuropsychological evaluations physicians use to diagnose dementia. Reassured that their minds are in fine shape, they lose the opportunity to benefit from early intervention. By the time such individuals actually demonstrate signs of frank dementia, they are beyond treatment. The brain pathology is so extensive that they decline more rapidly than other Alzheimer's patients, becoming helpless in a matter of months.

The roots of cognitive reserve appear to be established very early in life. Marcus Richards, a researcher at University College London, determined that childhood cognition—essentially, childhood IQ—was the greatest determinant of adult cognitive function. A high level of inherited intelligence helps, but just as important is early exposure to mentally stimulating activities. Yaakov Stern mentioned that he thought it would be interesting to track the cognitive health of people who had participated in the Head Start preschool program, to see whether their brains showed more resilience than a control group who had not benefited from such enrichment. I revealed my prejudices when I asked him if he thought that the current generation of children, who are more likely to plop down in front of a TV or chat via computer rather than ride their bikes, read books or enjoy real-life play with real-life peers, might exhibit less cognitive reserve as adults. To my surprise, he cited studies showing that video games, as well as messaging techniques that demand great dexterity on tiny keyboards, promoted certain types of cognitive development, although he had nothing to say for television.

RESTRICTED HORIZONS

Young people face strenuous mental challenges throughout the years they are in school, Stern pointed out. But the greatest hurdle—and the one that many people do not surmount—arrives in middle age, when the responsibilities of career and family become overwhelming, leaving little or no time remaining to pursue recreational activities. As people begin to notice deficits in memory and attention, their inclination is to adapt to restricted horizons. When plans for a family trip to the beach start to feel as complicated as Napoleon's preparations for his march on Russia, it's easier to scale back. People stop reading, relinquish hobbies and curtail social life in favor of familial responsibilities. They even choose an exercise routine that's a no-brainer, exchanging the challenge of a half-day weekend hike for twenty minutes of staring at a TV screen from the elliptical trainer. That we become novelty-averse is understandable, because most of what is "new" in midlife is frankly undesirable, a matter of contending with a sick parent, a depressed spouse or a troubled adolescent. What we want, most of all, is to maintain the status quo.

As children leave home and responsibilities lessen, some of us return to neuronally invigorating activities. I know many people in their late fifties, finally free, who are Googling long-lost friends, taking walking trips across the Pyrenees and embarking on new careers. I know just as many, however, who continue to feel constricted. They have a profound reluctance to alter the familiar outlines of their lives. These, notes Stern, are the ones who may find their cognitive reserve dangerously depleted. "Without a prospect," wrote Simone de Beauvoir, "a person's mind will grow crippled, hardened, sclerotic."

I was astonished when a couple I know, in their late fifties, informed me that under no circumstances could they ever eat dinner at 7:30 P.M. and attend a 9:40 movie, because they had to be tucked under the covers at 10:30 P.M., even on a Saturday night. "Embarrassing, but true," the husband wrote me in an e-mail. "It's scary, but very restful." I couldn't imagine that I'd ever find my horizons thus reduced, but I think of them when I find myself yawning uncontrollably while still in the shank of the evening.

Keeping the brain in fighting condition demands a combination of mental stimulation, physical activity and social interaction, and for many in midlife, all three are in short supply. Even occupations that are immensely challenging in the early years can grow repetitious and humdrum. "When it comes down to it," an attorney who had been handling real estate cases for his entire career told me, "they occasionally change the tax laws, and I have to catch up, but otherwise, at this point in my career, I've seen everything there is to see, and it's pretty tedious." Studies show that animals that learn new behaviors, and face new challenges every day, don't become senile at nearly the same rates as those who live in static environments. Because the brain demands novelty in order to build new synaptic connections, doing the same thing over and over again is a recipe for stagnation. And if you think that reading a junk paperback will satisfy those synaptic requirements, think again.

Before I actually sat down and totaled up the points, I figured I could claim a respectable level of cognitive reserve, enough to put me firmly in the black. There's no record of a childhood IQ test, which is not surprising—they were administered only under exceptional circumstances in the 1960s. If you include nursery school and kindergarten, I'd spent eighteen years in the academic arena. That was more than enough for me, but according to cognitive reserve theorists, I'd have to subtract some points for stopping with the B.A., since studies show that those who pursue advanced degrees build additional resilience.

I could give myself points for having a career as a journalist that was usually stimulating and happily free of busywork, but I'd lose some for the ten years I lost to unspecified brain fog, the bulk of which I spent at home rearing children. (In her 2005 book, *The Mommy Brain*, Katherine Ellison makes an excellent case for the mind-enhancing benefits of motherhood. Although I do not doubt that my presence at home greatly improved my offspring's level of cognitive reserve, I suspect that the extensive maternal perks Ellison described in her book wholly eluded me.) More points came off the total due to the likelihood I'd experienced mild traumatic brain injury. The years of insomnia, my natural inclination toward anxiety, my exposure to toxic substances, and my thyroid condition, which went untreated for so long, also snatched points away.

In the end, I realized that the balance sheet didn't look so great. In a 2005 study, published in the *American Journal of Epidemiology*, Constantine Lyketsos noted that the greatest cognitive benefits derived from participating in a range of activities, rather than single-mindedly applying oneself to one vocation. That was unfortunate, since my lone reserve-building activity involved the writing and research for this book. As my deadline grew closer, my exercise routine, once lively, had dwindled down to a few walks with the dogs each week. My social life wasn't much better—like most wives, I'm the one who makes those plans, and I had become more interested in the distribution of semicolons than the placement of guests around the dining table. I spent most days holed up in a little office with the shades down, exchanging the outside world for a view of my computer monitor. When I went home, I spent whatever mental energy I had left on my children. My husband knew better than to expect lively conversation. I realized that I'd let my life contract; I'd squeezed out many of the things that had once jazzed up my brain.

I told myself it was just temporary, a matter of needing to focus on finishing my book. But my existence wasn't going to flesh out unless I took action. I started thinking about the things I'd once loved and had put aside, one by one, in favor of adult responsibility and civic duty. There was horseback riding, spontaneous go-where-the-spirit-moves-you traveling, long-distance hiking and biking, cross-country skiing, fancy-pants cooking, darkroom photography, and performing in community theater, each of which offered its own special benefits to the brain. But who had time for any of it?

I checked in with my survey respondents, to see what they were doing to increase their cognitive reserve. I was hoping to hear that they were playing a lot of chess, which requires immense mental flexibility, planning and memory, especially if you play it blindfolded as some experts do. Not exactly. "I'm done learning," one man told me. "Now I just want to be entertained."

Fran's answer came shrieking back in e-mail.

"INVIGORATE MY BRAIN?" she wrote. "Isn't that something I'll do in retirement, when I'm old and have the time for crossword puzzles over coffee? I don't have time now. I barely have time to keep my leg muscles and heart in shape. I've yet to get to my arm muscles. Doesn't all that I have to remember to do count for anything?"

In their answers, some people mentioned brain-enhancing activities—mandatory hours on the StairMaster, regular tennis games or crack-of-dawn road biking, even guitar lessons, but always I detected guilt in their phrasing. Any minutes away from work or family were stolen, snatched from the hands of a teenager who really needed to learn to parallel-park before the big driving test. "As for the tennis," replied one woman who plays several days a week, "I'm not sure how useful it is. We have trouble keeping track of the score and usually have to retrace every point between the four of us."

Only one person, Victor, could say that he'd given the prospect any serious thought. "I'm always doing intellectual push-ups," he said. "Every year we hire a new crop of graduates, and I need to be able to communicate with them, so I challenge myself to learn new things. Recently, I taught myself a new programming language. I'm also a History Channel junkie, and I read a lot of nonfiction. I take at least two vacations a year involving new learning. I've gotten heavily involved with nonprofit advocacy groups, and I'm also beginning to teach. I wish I exercised my abs nearly as much."

BREAKING FREE

So, how to climb out of what had become a very deep rut? Charles Baxter, the novelist and essayist, now a professor at the University of Minnesota, wrote in an e-mail that he and his wife had moved to Minneapolis, "in part because the years were beginning to smear together and I wanted to do something that would jog the memory." Carly, who raises money for a major university, and her husband also moved, from her childhood home in New Haven to a small town on the outskirts of Boston. This, she suggests, may provide the ultimate cognitive challenge. "After knowing the same people for my entire life, every single thing I did was new, including my job, for which I needed to learn the names, positions and inclinations of my staff. I needed a new plumber and a new electrician. I didn't know who to call for anything. My children's teachers were all new, as were the kids' friends. I attribute most of my forgetfulness to this incessant novelty, but I don't doubt that it provided a huge jolt for a fiftyish brain. It might have been the best thing for us, although there were times when I was so profoundly confused that I wondered if we'd survive." George, whose mother suffered from Alzheimer's disease, explained that he'd switched careers, from building contractor to math teacher, "because it required more mental energy. I not only teach my math classes, but I enjoy working out math problems just for pleasure."

I decided to check out what other people were doing—short of moving house—to improve their levels of cognitive reserve. I was out in the real world, enjoying a couple of glasses of wine at a fund-raising event for 826 Valencia, a San Francisco organization that provides free writing classes for young people, when I met Richard Lang, fifty-six. More accurately, I met the structure that temporarily contained him. He was encased, from head to knees, in what upon closer examination turned out to be a jewel-encrusted "poetry jukebox." A cutout window at his eye level allowed him to maneuver through the crowd. "Pick a poem," he urged, "and I'll recite it for you."

"Well," I asked, "do you know the Billy Collins poem 'Forgetfulness'?"

He knew it, and he began to speak it as if it held great meaning for him. (If you'd like to read it yourself, you'll find it at the front of this book.)

Richard, who owns a lithography press just south of San Francisco, had begun memorizing poetry as a way of soothing himself after several difficult years. Both of his parents had died, he'd had a couple of car accidents and cancer surgery. His house had burned down, and, understandably, he found it impossible to sleep. He began by memorizing a poem by Wallace Stevens called "Sunday Morning."

"I took my time with it," he said, "and I really dropped into the meaning of it. It was a great palliative to insomnia, for that time at 3:15 A.M., when the bedroom turns into the switching yard for the freight trains of anxiety." When he had memorized sixty poems, his wife, artist Judith Selby, constructed the poetry jukebox and presented it to him as a gift. "Eventually," he said, "I learned a hundred and four poems, and it became a party trick, but to me, it has always been more than that. The images in a poem form a ladder in my mind. In order to recall them, I need to think about how one thing leads to another. I find that I've extended that practice to the rest of my life. I'm more aware of how things are connected to each other, and it makes it somewhat easier for me to recall what it is I'm supposed to do, and where, and why."

Surely, memorizing poetry was excellent mental exercise and an interesting option in my quest to build cognitive reserve. I could join my father in his out-of-the-blue recitations of Kipling's "Gunga Din," which was one of his favorites. " 'You may talk o' gin and beer, / When you're quartered safe out here,' " he'd roar, and everybody would shut up and listen.

But if I wished to maximize my efforts, perhaps reciting poetry was too sedentary. Unless I really got into the accompanying dramatic gestures, I'd still need more physical exercise. Studies were rolling in faster than I could read them that pointed to the immediate and long-term benefits to be gained from specific types of exertion. Aerobic exercise pumped additional blood to the brain, delivering oxygen and glucose. The body responded by building new capillaries, and by boosting brain-protective chemicals, such as BDNF, that help strengthen neuronal connections. An investigation executed by University of Illinois professor Arthur Kramer revealed that a group of elderly people who participated in aerobic fitness showed significant improvement in executive function, planning, scheduling and multitasking, but that another group, engaged in strength and flexibility training, showed no such effects. Several new studies demonstrate that those who engage in physical activity just twice a week have a 60 percent lower chance of developing Alzheimer's disease. According to Miia Kivipelto, an investigator at the Karolinska Institute, the benefit is even more pronounced among individuals who are ApoE4 carriers.

Fred Gage, who you may remember as the scientist who pointed out to the world that neurogenesis occurred in the adult brain, corroborated Kramer's findings in 2005, and upped the ante. In a study published in *Neuroscience,* he revealed that mice that started exercising in old age—about nineteen months—were able to reduce the typical age-related slowdown of the growth of new neurons. After the mice ran voluntarily on the wheel for a month (I imagined rodents in tiny Nike running suits, long pink tails streaming), they boasted a whopping 50 percent increase in new neurons compared to the amount they generated when sedentary. Gage noted that a group of more youthful mice that exercised regularly showed the greatest neuron growth of all groups, a finding that suggests that a similar effect might be present in humans in midlife.

When I saw a picture in *Health* magazine of Nan Wiener, a fifty-three-year-old magazine editor who lives in San Francisco, looking as if she was having the time of her life as she danced with a young and handsome partner, I got an idea. I'd just read a study that found ballroom dancing reduced the risk of developing dementia by 76 percent. Lead investigator Joe Verghese, a researcher at Albert Einstein School of Medicine, showed that the demands of dancing—remembering the steps, moving in precise time to the music and adapting your movements to your partner's—afforded considerable protection, presumably by building cognitive reserve. The results Verghese obtained suggested that it was better mental exercise than learning a language or a musical instrument, or doing crossword puzzles, or taking a class that required study or memorization.

All of this was news to Nan. She'd fallen in love with salsa seven years earlier, and except for the year after she'd slipped in her kitchen and broken her ankle, she'd been dancing once or twice a week in classes and clubs ever since. Her husband, a music critic, was quite happy to remain at home with their daughter and let her get her exercise. "It's actually a great hobby to have, if you have young kids," she observed. "You don't go out until after they've gone to sleep, so it doesn't eat into family time too much." Dancing half the night away did gobble up hours of sleep, but the energy rush she got from learning a new step or dancing with a talented partner made it worthwhile.

We agreed to meet in Sausalito, at Horizons, a bar-restaurant on the bay that is usually overrun with tourists. On this particular evening, however, Horizons was hosting a well-known salsa band, and the crowd that usually turned up at her other haunts—the Allegra Ballroom in Emeryville and Jelly's, near the baseball stadium—was heading this way.

Nan was bright-eyed and extremely fit, attired in sleek black jeans, heels and a dressy blouse. At Horizons, we paid our cover charge and walked into the bar, which was already jammed. In seconds, I developed a terminal case of wallflower awkwardness. The last time I'd been to such a venue with a female friend, I was in my twenties.

"What happens here?" I whispered. "Do you have to stand around and wait for a guy to ask you to dance?"

Before she could reply, Nan was gone, swept into the arms of a powerfully built young man whose head was adorned with short perky twists. From their animated chat, I gathered that she knew him from other salsa parties. They were instantly in synch, both displaying an impressive grasp of the difficult-to-master ability to wiggle your hips relentlessly while you keep your upper body perfectly still. They whirled apart and came back together, feet constantly moving in tiny little steps.

"Yes!" I thought. "This is for me!" If I could learn salsa and merengue and maybe a sexy tango—and stockpile neuronal connections at the same time—I was definitely up for Intervention #10.

The next morning, I called a dancing school in San Francisco that specialized in salsa lessons and learned that if I showed up on Monday night at seven-thirty, with ten bucks and a pair of leather-soled shoes, I'd be just in time to start a new session. The instructor, Evan Margolin, directed us to form a half dozen lines that stretched across the room, so that he could teach us some steps. There was a lot to think about. I had to listen to the music, stay in time, remember the steps, concentrate on what the instructor was saying and, most important, refrain from crashing into my partner, or anybody else. Zoning out was definitely not an option. Within a half hour, I felt something shift. I no longer needed to count out loud, or attend to every single beat. Some new synaptic connections had obviously been made: My body knew what it was doing.

By the second session, we were into some very demanding footwork that I couldn't remember for more than two seconds. It was at times like these that I recognized the scope of my deficit of working memory. "Concentrate," I hissed at myself. "Listen to the teacher." It was harder than I could have anticipated.

After I completed six sessions, I felt moderately salsa-ready. I sent a bunch of e-mails to some local pals, explaining that it was possible to boost your cognitive reserve and drink a margarita at the same time. Just around then, research emerged from McGill University showing that tango dancing was likely even better for the brain than salsa. There were more elements involved: the forward, backward, side-to-side weight shift, the one-legged stance, walking forward and backward in a straight line and turning in a narrow space. Now, all I needed was a middle-aged Argentinian dance partner, and I'd be all set. I recommended to my friends that we go to Jelly's, where they offered lessons early in the evening, before the real action began. I might as well have suggested that we all go bungee jumping. A few of the women were game, but their husbands flatly refused. I played the cognitive-reserve angle for all it was worth, but I had no takers. This segment of my memory-hungry crowd was evidently getting their nourishment elsewhere.

BACK TO SCHOOL

Survey respondents noted that they knew going back to school would be good for their brains, but doubts about their ability to absorb and retain new information made them reluctant to take up a language or begin to study a musical instrument. Although few studies have been executed to assess the benefits of such training in midlife, both music and language learning have been found to enhance visual and verbal memory, as well as IQ, in children. One investigation, conducted by researchers from the University of Florida, examined the effect of individualized piano instruction on executive function in a group of adult volunteers, all of whom were novices. On neuropsychological tests given before and after three months of training, specific improvements were noted in working memory, planning, concentration and the ability to select a strategy and stick with it.

Jacob, a magazine editor who began to study guitar seriously in his midforties, told me that it was easier than he expected. "I think that when I sit myself down quietly, I have much more focus than I had as a child," he observed, "although my memory is just as bad as it ever was. What I've learned from studying guitar is that my fingers have a memory of their own. I can feel something happening in my brain, as the fingering becomes automatic. So when I practice something, even though it doesn't make sense at first, I know that repeating it ad nauseum will help me to master it. Of course, that mastery might only be good for the day—I could completely forget it. But I can pick it up again, with only a little effort."

Grace, whose two children are talented musicians, joked that after her profound involvement in twelve years of violin lessons, she'd expected to be able to pick up the instrument and play it perfectly. In reality, she didn't have the requisite dexterity. Recently, at fifty-eight, she began to study piano. She echoed Jacob's sentiments: "When I sit down and put my mind to it, I'm much less distracted than I was at seventeen, when my heart and energy were elsewhere. I think I've been able to compensate for whatever brain-cell death occurred along the way. To me, learning an instrument is unlike anything else I've ever taken on. It requires not only that I learn something in an intellectual way, but that the learning is absorbed by my body, by my fingers and hands and foot, so that I can read the music and interpret what it is telling me to do and do it, instantaneously. I've had to become aware of what my fingers are doing, of where my hands are on the piano, without looking at them. I can practically feel new synaptic connections in the making as I get better at it."

Nan—and Jacob and Grace and Richard Lang, aka the poetry jukebox—confirmed what I'd sensed: that it was entirely possible to boost your level of cognitive reserve while having a rollicking good time. In midlife, especially, we did not need to bore ourselves half to death with memory exercises. There were a million far more entertaining alternatives.

I encountered a handful of midlife adults who took the idea of continuing their education so seriously that they boldly enrolled in law school and medical school. Each of them realized, from the beginning, that it would be a serious error to pretend that they had the same capacities as traditional students. In some areas, they were much weaker, but in others, they found unexpected strengths.

Dawn Swanson, now fifty, was forty when she decided that she'd worked long enough as a nursing-home operator. She'd always wanted to be a doctor, but when she gave birth to her first child, at seventeen, she told me, "It nearly ended the dream for good." At forty-three, she left her job and enrolled in an undergraduate degree program at a local college. "I'd never heard of age-associated memory impairment," she told me, "so I didn't factor it in. I just knew that I had three kids at home, and I'd never been the sharpest knife in the block, so I was going to have to study all the time."

The young students in her classes crammed for exams, leaving their studying to the night before. "When they walked into the test," she said, "they appeared to know everything. But the moment they walked out, they forgot every word of it." She organized study groups that met two or three times a week. "We just kept drilling on it, until it made it into long-term memory," she said.

Dawn realized that her greatest asset was her ability to step back and put things in perspective. "I was very good at seeing how ideas linked together," she explained, "and that allowed me to make connections and draw inferences. Still, I was painfully slow. The teacher would explain a concept in algebra, and the kids would get it instantly. I'd be mulling it over and over. But those same kids were the ones who failed the final, because nothing really sank in."

Around the time she completed her undergraduate credits and applied to medical school, her husband asked her for a divorce. "He was desperately opposed to my decision," she said. In an effort to save money, she did her own legal work. Her inability to hang on to the facts during the four days of the divorce proceedings made her wonder if her application to med school was a mistake. "My anxiety level was sky-high," she said. "I was under extreme stress, pumping tons of cortisol—I call that the 'forgetting' drug—and there was plenty of information I couldn't access. Although I went over the legal documents again and again, I just couldn't make them stick."

She applied exclusively to schools in Mexico and the Caribbean. According to Dawn, it's virtually impossible to get into an American medical school as a "nontraditional student." "The AMA wants you to be around to practice for at least fifty years, so people who are already in their forties are not really candidates," she explained.

When she was accepted to the program at Guadalajara, she packed up her life, sent her middle child off to college two years early, and convinced her ex-husband that it would be a learning experience for her youngest child to accompany her. "I was one of about eighty Americans, most of whom were at least in their thirties," she told me, "which was sort of a relief. I knew they'd have similar issues, and that we could work through them together."

One of her fellow students was a dentist who had retired at sixty-five and promptly applied to med school. Another was an air force pilot who had four grown children, all of them superstars. He wanted to become a psychiatrist. "What we all discovered," Dawn explained, "is that working memory is handy dandy, but getting through medical school is really about long-term consolidation and reasoning. You need to have a flowchart in your mind that leads you to the answer. You realize that there are patterns to everything—life experience has shown you that. Basically, you're using the same technique that as an adult allows you to meet a new person and know immediately with whom you are dealing—you've seen it before, and you'll see it again. Sometimes there was material I couldn't access—a formula, for instance—but I understood the concept, and so I could build on it."

In her second year of med school, Dawn's identical twin sister, a diabetic, died of a heart attack. "I had to do everything in my power to bring my stress levels down," she said, "because I couldn't remember anything. I exercised a lot. I taped everything, and I'd go out walking with the earphones. I walked and read a book at the same time.

"People want an excuse not to succeed," said Dawn, who finished medical school in 2003, completed her internship in a family practice near Spokane, Washington, and is on track to complete her residency in 2007. "I wondered if I'd be able to handle being on call all the time. That's considered an appropriate job for a twenty-five-year-old. I figured with so little sleep, my memory would be wrecked. But then I understood that what was a new experience for young interns—having to stay up round the clock to care for other people—I'd been doing for over twenty years. Mothers are on call twenty-four hours a day. And there's no one to take over your shift when you're caring for a sick kid by yourself, never mind two or three of them.

"I actually think my short-term memory is better now than it was when I was younger and I had small kids running around. I'm very focused. I have a lot more energy. I know what I'm capable of doing, and I'm acutely aware of the danger spots, because I can't afford to screw up. I don't try to carry unnecessary things around in my head. What does it prove, really, if you can remember a shopping list?

"I'm not interested in excuses, although I sure had enough of them. I was the first in my class to pass the boards. It helped that I had my kids. They were my greatest supporters, and many times, they were the only ones. I was not going to let them down. Without them, I might never have done it."

WORDSMITHS

Unless you were somewhere other than the western world during July 2003, it was impossible to escape the news. Joe Verghese, the Albert Einstein College of Medicine researcher who studied ballroom dancing, produced results showing that people who solved crossword puzzles four days a week had a 47 percent lower chance of developing dementia than those who only tackled the puzzles occasionally.

When the word got out, crossword puzzles were suddenly hot. So was Sudoku, a number placement puzzle that was newly in vogue. Sidney, a publishing executive, fifty-five, reported that he'd begun to do crosswords during his morning train commute to the city. "Like most semieducated people my age," he wrote, "I can finish Monday and Tuesday in twenty minutes, and lately, I've even gotten Wednesday and the occasional Thursday. Friday, I don't bother. I don't have the patience for the Sunday puzzle. I go through the easy ones, but usually I leave it at that."

There were times, he confided, that the crossword brought him more angst than satisfaction. "This morning," he wrote me in an e-mail, "the clue was 'presidential middle name.' So I started to run the list of presidents backward. Unfortunately, I got stuck after George Bush. Although I could visualize Bill Clinton, his name eluded me for a minute or more, a long time for someone who is accustomed to handling tons of obscure information. In that moment, fear arose. I thought it was a surefire case of incipient Alzheimer's."

I admitted to Sidney that the fact that he could solve puzzles at all was impressive to me. "I can't manage," I told him. "I think it's the whole visuospatial thing. Just looking at them makes my head swim.

I can't keep in mind the configurations of words and letters." I suspected that success at crosswords required a specific type of mind—one that easily amassed and held quantities of what I called trivia, and others referred to as factual information. It seemed clear, as well, that you needed a large amount of working memory at your disposal. If, like me, you could barely recall the clue for ten down long enough to locate the squares on the page, you were in trouble.

I called Will Shortz, the fifty-three-year-old editor of the *New York Times* crossword puzzle. He's been creating puzzles since he designed his own major in enigmatology—the science of puzzle construction—at Indiana University. I asked him what he thought of Joe Verghese's pronouncement. Had his page of the daily paper become attractive to high-paying advertisers?

Nothing much had changed in the paper, he explained, but subscriptions to the *New York Times* online crossword puzzle, available for a year for $39.95, were selling like crazy. He'd always known that crossword puzzles were tops for building mental flexibility. "They're an all-around mental workout," he said enthusiastically. "They tap different parts of the brain, testing knowledge of all sorts of things—things you learned in school, what's going on in the world now, in films, sports, current events. You have to be flexible, in order to look at a clue and see the many ways in which it can lead, because puzzles are full of puns, tricks and deceptions. They're great for cross-training your brain."

I asked him what kind of personalities were particularly good puzzle solvers. "You have to love words, of course," he said. "But the person who is really good usually has a very mathematical sort of mind, which allows him or her to see how the words might lock into a grid."

"Ah," I said, beginning to understand why I had never had much success. (Soon after I interviewed Shortz, *Wordplay*, a documentary about his career as an enigmatologist came out. Much of the film was shot at Shortz's annual crossword tournament held in Stamford, Connecticut. The usual solving skills are not enough to get you to the top in Stamford. You also have to be rocket fast. Many people—middle-aged and a great deal older, who'd attended for decades—peered into the camera, but the champion was—you guessed it—a twenty-year-old puzzling prodigy still in college.)

Shortz directed me to the *New York Times* Puzzle Forum message board, where he assured me that I would find more crossword aficionados than I could handle. I posted a brief message, asking if anyone had taken up "solving," as they refer to it, for the express purpose of improving memory and attention.

Within an hour, my mailbox was stuffed with replies. One man noted that even though he was a champion puzzler—one who competed in the annual American Crossword Puzzle Tournament directed by Will Shortz—it hadn't helped him with his main problem—his prosopagnosia. I wasn't surprised that he knew the right word for being unable to recognize people you know fairly well.

The response that resonated most, however, came from Courtenay "Co" Crocker, fifty-six. The CEO of a metal-fabrication company, he'd been an occasional crossword solver throughout his life, but puzzles had recently helped him get through some very unhappy times. Six years earlier, when his daughter was diagnosed with leukemia, he spent an enormous amount of time in her hospital room and waiting with her before procedures.

"I was only fifty years old, for heaven's sake," he wrote in his e-mail, "but I was forgetting birthdays, meetings, people's names, what I was doing and, very often, where I was going. I am sure I was hypersensitive to my memory loss, as my dad, at the same time, was suffering the debilitating effects of advanced Alzheimer's disease." He began to take puzzles with him to the hospital. While his daughter slept, he solved them, one right after the other.

"Very late one night, I drew a six-by-six grid on a blank sheet of paper," he noted, "and I started filling in words, constructing for the first time a puzzle of my own. I thought that the more puzzles I solved, the better I would be at constructing, so I set about the task with vigor, taking on eight to ten puzzles a day. Although my constructing ability didn't improve significantly, my mind seemed sharper and more focused. I can attest that if you exercise the mind with these sorts of mental gymnastics, it can be trained toward lucidity." When Co finally constructed a puzzle that made him proud, he shipped it off to Will Shortz, who selected it for publication in the *New York Times* on June 23, 2005. "It was a tremendous thrill," acknowledged Co, "to see my puzzle up in lights."

As you've seen, mental stimulation and physical activity go a long way toward establishing high levels of cognitive reserve, but the third factor—social interaction—is every bit as important. When people interact with others, basic processes such as working memory, speed of processing and verbal knowledge come into play. All the senses are tapped—vision, hearing, touch, and even smell, noted University of Michigan scientist Oscar Ybarra, who found a close relationship between how much social contact people reported and how well they did when asked to perform a variety of neuropsychological tests. Laura Fratiglioni, from the Stockholm Gerontology Research Centre at the Karolinska Institute, completed a study that demonstrated the importance of social involvement, which in the group she observed reduced the risk of dementia by 40 percent.

"You may not realize it," said Duke's Lawrence Katz, the late scientist who, soon after our interview, sent me blindfolded through my own front door, "but social interaction is way down. We've taken to sending e-mails to the office next door. It's now considered quite intrusive to telephone or to show up in person if it is possible to e-mail, and that's a real sociological switch. There's very little reason to get together in person, which limits our ability to create new associations. But the more new associations we can build, the more we activate synapses, and the more BDNF we produce, so this is definitely a catch-22. The stronger and richer the network of associations, the more the brain is protected.

"We're actually deceiving ourselves, with all this talk about how well connected the Internet has allowed us to become. The single best thing you can do for your brain is to just be around other people in a meaningful way. That doesn't mean just working with people—it means genuine face-to-face-interactions. If I showed you a picture of what your brain was doing when you were involved with another person, you wouldn't believe it. There are specialized areas that are just devoted to this. And the absence of human interaction is just deadly for the brain."

Edward Hallowell, the psychiatrist who specializes in ADHD, noted that disconnectedness is a lethal danger. "You need a plan to make sure you stay genuinely connected with living humans you know and like," he wrote in his latest book, *CrazyBusy*. "Easy? Just count the number of minutes you spend each day with live human beings, in person. . . . Compare that number with, say, twenty years ago or even ten." He observed that human moments, to a large extent, have been replaced with electronic moments. "People spend less time in each other's physical presence. Family dinners, face-to-face conversations, and live meetings have been replaced by eating alone, by conversing on the cell phone or by IM and by teleconferences. The electronic moment is hugely efficient, rapid and easy. However, the human moment conveys far more information: tone of voice, body language, facial expression, and all the nonverbal cues that constitute such a vital part of human communication." In 1960, 40 percent of people who were sixty-five and older lived in the home of an adult child. By the late 1990s, this number had dropped to 4 percent. When you consider that 71 percent of seniors over the age of sixty-five in the United States live alone, and many spend more than seven hours a day without any social contact, perhaps the rate at which they succumb to Alzheimer's disease should not come as a surprise.

I was thinking about that while I drove up the steep hill to the house in Larkspur where the Dannenburgs have lived for forty-one years. Zvi, the eighty-year-old firecracker, had invited me over to meet his wife, Marjorie, who at eighty-two was still running her home-repair business. "She drives a pickup and she does plumbing, wiring and light carpentry," he said. "Recently, she replaced a toilet by herself. I guess she didn't feel like waiting for help."

When I arrived, I chatted with Marjorie for a few minutes, but I could tell that Zvi couldn't wait to take me down to his "little empire," the room in which he maintained his music. We exited the kitchen, clambered down some challenging stairs, crossed a rocky stretch of backyard, and entered the little empire, where the walls were lined, floor to ceiling, with record albums and CDs. He'd discovered most of his recordings in thrift stores, and he still toured Salvation Army outlets and musical specialty stores all over the Bay Area. He spent at least three hours every day in his empire, listening to music and studying liner notes. Cataloguing so much music was a great deal of work, he said. "But I've got it so that I can put my hands on almost anything in a few seconds," he noted, selecting a CD from a shelf and extracting the liner notes. "You see this?" he asked, pointing to a name in a tiny font. I noticed that he didn't need eyeglasses. "I was talking to a fellow on the jogging path the other day, and I realized from what he told me about his father, who had just passed away, that he must have been the first violinist in this orchestra. So I'm going to give him the CD as a gift. I really respond to music with all my being," he said. "Every molecule in my body vibrates."

After that visit, I didn't see Zvi for a few months. I was out on the path again when I spotted his crooked blue hat, way off in the distance. I broke into an uncharacteristic jog, surprising the dogs, and hoped that before I reached him, I'd somehow manage to remember his wife's name. "Cathryn! Not Cathleen," he shouted when he saw me. "And Rosie, and Radar! And how is your son doing with the math tutor? And how is it going now with your book?"

"You're astounding," I said when I reached him, and planted a kiss on his cheek.

"Well," he answered, "you know my secret. I'm too busy to get old."

CONCLUSION

• • •

I know what you're thinking. You're trying to decide which interventions might work for you. Maybe you've already gone to your
supermarket and come away with vitamins and supplements, now
forming a conga line on your kitchen counter. Perhaps you've signed
up for mindfulness meditation or, like Nan Wiener, you've booked
your salsa lessons. Maybe you've gone out and bought a fat book of
crossword puzzles, or, like Bill McGlynn, you're already a serious fan
of MyBrainTrainer.

On the other hand, you might just be sitting there wondering how
it all turned out for me. Did I wind up in a different state of mind?

It's a fair question. People ask me all the time if I'm "better," and
honestly, I can say that I am. This doesn't mean that I don't occasionally run a Grand Trifecta of Forgetfulness. Recently, I drove into the
city without my wallet or my cell phone, both of which remained at
home on my desk. I scraped around in the bottom of my purse to
come up with 50 cents for the meter. Lunch was out of the question.
I didn't find out until I returned home that my elder son was speed-
dialing me. That was just as well: I'd also forgotten to have pizza delivered to his high school for a noon meeting of the government club.

I apologized, of course. Then I pointed out that, evidently, he had a perfectly good dialing finger, and next time he might consider using it to arrange delivery of his own pizza by ordering it the night before.

These all-out festivals of forgetting used to be the rule. Now, they're a rarity.

Although it would be immensely satisfying to tell you which of the ten interventions did the trick, I can't. I'm not surprised: From the beginning, I knew that the flaws in my "make myself a guinea pig" methodology, which involved pursuing multiple, overlapping research protocols, would muddy my results. In truth, there was no other way. Even if I'd had ten years—one for each intervention—I would not have been able to say, for sure, that my thyroid medication made the difference, and that the vitamins and supplements did nothing at all, because the most crucial variable—the physiology of the brain—end-lessly rearranges itself in response to environmental and biochemical factors. Eat less trans fat? Different brain. Dance your ass off three nights a week? Different brain, yet again.

Nonetheless, the answer is, "Yes, I'm better." I take the vitamins and supplements. When I need to, I swallow Provigil, which I prefer to regard as a mental tool, rather than a crutch. I'm planning more neurofeedback sessions, which I believe hold promise for those who wish to improve their attention and focus. Despite the careful atten-tion Richard Shames paid to my thyroid gland and Tracy Kuo's best efforts at the Stanford Sleep Disorder Center, I'm still a short, ineffi-cient sleeper. I know that getting "the sleep thing handled" is essential for making the most of my cognitive function, but for me it remains a work in progress. In a few weeks, I'll head back down to Palo Alto to be wired up for that sleep study. It will provide the most intimate look possible at what my brain does in bed, and hopefully, some answers.

I cannot pinpoint the thing that made the difference, but I know the fog has lifted—instead of the equivalent of the impenetrable white stuff that tumbles in off the Pacific, blanketing the Golden Gate Bridge every summer afternoon, most days my fog is light, no heavier than the wispy smoke from a cottage chimney. That, I can manage. These days, I find I'm attentive to moments that might otherwise slip away. Last summer, I sat cross-legged on the beach, my lanky younger son folded into my lap, feeling nostalgia in advance: Very soon, he wouldn't fit. Consciously, I made a memory—his smell, his streaked and salty hair, the color and warmth of his skin, the roughness of the sand on his back. The moment's mine forever—but only because I took the time to secure it.

I have found that the answer lies in acknowledging the problem. This sounds simple, but it is not, because it also means that you must acknowledge the fact that, like it or not, you are getting older. You can't slap off your mistakes like so many mosquitoes, or stick your head in the sand. Nor can you generalize, and blame "your terrible memory," because, as you now realize, there's a great deal more to it than that. You must be willing to dissect the "anatomy of a fuckup" as carefully as you explored the innards of that frog in biology class. Once you find out where you went wrong, you can classify it. Was it a matter of sleep deprivation? A question of having forgotten to eat lunch? A bona fide hippocampal failure? Get the facts, and you will automatically alter your behavior, which in my experience will help you avoid making the same error the next time around. You really have no choice. Unless you are willing to take the time to get to the root of your problem, all the list making and Post-it note sticking will not help. Inevitably, you'll leave your lists behind. And the extensive Post-it collection on your office door will serve as abstract art and nothing more.

My counteroffensive was quite effective. In time, I got my mojo back—ideas meshed, names made themselves readily available and words flew from my brain to my fingers to the monitor screen. Slowly, I worked my way back to a mind I could trust. It meant an end to wishful thinking, to pretending that one day I'd wake up without any deficits. For the remainder of my life, I'd have to acknowledge my weaknesses. To insist upon doing things the same way I had always done them was as much a vanity as refusing to wear reading glasses and making other people read me the menu. I'd need to apply fail-safe strategies to every aspect of my work and family life. There could be no procrastination. There was no such place, I recognized, as "the back of my mind." There could be no guessing, because I was always wrong. And sadly, there would be no multitasking, ever. In midlife, I'd learned my lesson. If I flew by the seat of my pants even briefly, I could expect to spend hours cleaning up the detritus from the inevitable crash.

If that sounds like an inflexible, ascetic way to live, in practice it is not. It is easier and in many ways liberating to know that if I really expect to return my son's pants to Macy's, I need to do more than think about it. I'm going to have to put the white bag with the big red star in the car, not in the trunk, but in the front seat. Once the trousers are there, beside me, I am free to turn my attention to more significant things. There is no need to remind myself, every time I drive past the mall, that, stupidly, I have forgotten them again.

Over the many months of my research, I sensed that one day, sometime in the future, I wouldn't care so much. Although many essential cognitive skills—for instance, the ability to remember names or recognize faces—decline precipitously as the decades go by, people's self-reported impressions reflect a different understanding. "Asked how they would describe their memories," said clinical psychologist Thomas Crook, who studies the subject, "people who are in their forties are the most critical. In their fifties, they feel a little bit better about their capacities, and by the time they reach their sixties, they're as satisfied as they were in their early thirties."

Why was that? Matthew, an attorney in his sixties, tried to explain it to me. "I'm past worrying about it," he said. "If I were in my forties, trying to do my job, I know it would really bother me. It depends on where you are in your life. But I'm getting near retirement. And to me, it's just another sign that I need to think about doing different things. I need to stop hanging on. It's a far more desperate feeling earlier."

When he spoke those words, I looked at him closely. He wasn't kidding around. Here was a man who was smart as hell. His remarkable cognitive abilities had provided a handsome livelihood for nearly four decades. Unlike some people, he wasn't in denial—he acknowledged that he wasn't as sharp and he wasn't as fast. But neither was he frantic. To him, this was simply part of the ebb and the flow that made for the tide of life. He and his wife were enjoying the process of simplifying their existence. Their children were grown and gone. The frantic years of midlife were already at a close. No longer was there a need to divide their attention in a million ways. Matt and his wife were hardly destined for a golf cart retirement. He was trying to determine which of several nonprofit organizations' boards he would join.

I thought about Matt often as I finished writing this book. I knew that he was a tough lawyer, the kind of guy who never settled for anything short of the most he could get. And yet, he was at peace with what he saw as a natural transition. At what point might I stop dwelling on what had been lost, I wondered, and begin to relish what I had gained with age? For Matt, at least, perspective and insight, fused with acceptance, formed the cornerstone of wisdom. The rest, presumably, he could get from Google.

ACKNOWLEDGMENTS

. . .

Knowing just how fickle my memory can be, I started keeping this list long before I began writing. In retrospect, that was a smart move. I had no idea how lengthy it would become. Looking back, I'm awed and moved by the numbers of people who contributed their time, their skills and their love and support.

Thanks to my agent, Suzanne Gluck, and her diligent staff at William Morris. I feel immensely lucky to have her on my side of the negotiating table. My gratitude to my extraordinary book editor, Gail Winston. Calm, decisive, deft and smart, she has an uncanny understanding of this writer's psyche, knowing when to push and when to praise, and when to drop everything and head out for a long lunch or a little time in Saks. Thanks to others at HarperCollins—Rachel Elinsky, Tina Andreadis, Jamie Brickhouse, Julie Elmuccio and Sarah Whitman-Salkin. Huge thanks to Camille McDuffie, whose company, Goldberg McDuffie, graciously presented *Carved in Sand* to the media, and to the enthusiastic Steve Bennett, whose company, AuthorBytes, designed the Web site.

Under the circumstances I've described in these pages, you might reasonably wonder how I managed to write a book, especially one of such inherent complexity. Had I not learned to delegate, it would have been impossible. The universe bestowed upon me a multitude of gifts. Among them was Elizabeth Crane, who functions as my spare brain. Anything that there is a possibility that I'll forget (and that's quite a lot, as you know), I toss onto one of her many spinning plates. We have many uplifting exchanges each week, but the one that sticks with me came in the form of a reply to a frantic e-mail, on a day when forgetfulness reigned. I'd ended my message, "Losing it." Her reply was brief: "Keeping it." That said it all.

It is an odd truth that today you can work with people intimately for years—while they're hundreds of miles away. That's how it worked with another member of my team, researcher Cathy Dunn. I met her once, for lunch in Los Angeles, but from that moment forward, it was e-mail all the way. If a brick wall stood between me and my grasp of some concept, simple or arcane, Dunn would provide an explanation, often within minutes of the moment she received my e-mail query. In three years, I believe I stumped her once. Each month, she forwarded me a thick research packet, stuffed with news from professional journals. I knew for a fact that if it was important, I'd find it in those pages.

Elisha Yang, a senior from Tamalpais High School, flawlessly managed the hundreds of books that the Marin County Free Library system dutifully delivered, fetching and returning, recording copyright information, and standing for hours over a copying machine. Talleah Bridges helped gather data, as did Roxane Assaf and Melanie Haiken. Jan Stoner provided early support and long-term encouragement, as did Catherine Valeriote. Ben Winter's admirable company, Letter Perfect Transcription, turned hundreds of hours of digital recordings into neatly typed interviews, almost as fast as I could e-mail the files. And then, although it seems somehow improper to thank an inanimate object, there was the Olympus digital recorder itself, a gleaming device about half the size of my palm, that allowed me to keep track of hundreds of interviews, initiating playback right from my computer's desktop. Equally crucial and deserving of praise is Thesaurus.com, that online repository of all the words that played hide-and-seek when I needed them most.

There must be people who write books in a vacuum, freed from the ordinary requirements of life, like laundry, cooking and homework, but I am definitely not one of them. Those who stepped in to help in this capacity deserve enormous praise: Delmy Arevalo and Mark and Pam Chavez come immediately to mind. They were always ready to help, showering my family with love and smiles, making it possible for me to sustain some very long stints at the keyboard.

And then there are the Writer Friends, without whom it would have been quite impossible to get through a day. I owe a debt of gratitude to Jason Roberts, author of *A Sense of the World*, who helped me solve countless "insurmountable" literary problems, even when he had a toddler on his knee, an infant in his arms and his own book to get to press. I'm equally indebted to Michelle Slatalla, author of *The Town on Beaver Creek*, who listened for hours over lunch at Toast, our local hangout. Bravely, she took on the task of reading an early draft, not to mention the preparation and hosting of two Thanksgiving dinners with her husband, Josh Quittner. I offer the heartiest thanks—and hopes for many more hours of professional and personal camaraderie. Thanks as well to Katherine Ellison, author of *The Mommy Brain*, who was willing and able to talk neuroscience. I'm grateful to Alan Deutschman, author of *Change or Die*, who generously set me on this path with a couple of well-placed e-mails, and nurtured this project from infancy to maturity. Nor can I leave out Jeffrey Trachtenberg, who helped me grasp the intricacies of book marketing, or his wife, Elizabeth Sanger, who has been talking sense into me since we worked together at Barron's, some twenty-five years ago. Thanks as well to Andrew Solomon, author of *The Noonday Demon*, whose e-mailed advice, often arriving from far corners of the globe, proved extraordinarily valuable. Thanks, also, to Jody Winer for her invaluable proofreading skills. Finally, I must express my gratitude to Carolyn Meyer, who has shown me, over nearly three decades, what it means to be a working writer.

And then there are the magazine editors, whose kind attentions have shaped my work. My thanks to Ilena Silverman and Vera Titunik at the *New York Times Magazine*, who published "In Search of Lost Time," an article that outlined the ideas that eventually grew into this book. To write for Titunik and Silverman is to learn, finally, what good is: They prune away at what you think is your finest work, and demand better, until one day, it is all there and just as it should be. Then, if you are very lucky, you are placed in the capable hands of Renee Michael, fact-checker extraordinaire, who teaches you what it means to be accurate. My thanks as well to Liz Brody, editor at *O, The Oprah Magazine*, for her careful work on my feature story about the cognitive side effects of antidepressant drugs, the research for which provided the seeds for Chapter 15, "What Your Doctor Forgot to Tell You." Other editors from years long past also deserve thanks: Peter Herbst, Betsy Carter, Michelle Stacey, Judith Daniels and Jane Amsterdam among them.

And then there are the guestroom friends and relatives, those who graciously offered me their hospitality whenever I blew into town to conduct interviews or do research. Thanks to Tom and Amy Jakobson, Stacey Spector, Margaret and Alan Metcalf-Klaw, Jim Wilson and Janet Shur, Julie and Jeremy Levy, Cindy Albert-Link and Carol Hopkins, for their comfy beds and well-laid tables, but mostly for their willingness to deal with my midnight pacings and requests for directions and rides.

My appreciation to the members of my extended family, who put up with missed birthday parties and holiday celebrations, not to mention last-minute cancellations of the best-laid plans. They found time for me whenever I could sandwich them in between appointments. Thanks, especially, to my parents-in-law, Sid and Gloria Ramin, who showed indefatigable interest and pride in all aspects of the project, to my mother and father, and to my aunt, Helen Mintz, who regularly e-mailed me bits of amusement, advice and comfort. Thanks to friends who have become part of the family, especially to Diane and Gary Tsyporin and their son, Jeremy, who helped out in innumerable ways. Thanks to my sister-in-law, Lisa Jakobson, who turned her camera's big lens on me and produced the jacket photo and many of the pictures on my Web site.

Thanks, as well, to Pat Carroll Marasco, who made sure that

the research team actually got paid and the electricity and phone service stayed on, and to Kim Holmes, whose bodywork program prevented me from developing incapacitating occupational illnesses like carpal tunnel syndrome, writer's elbow and author's hunch. Thanks, also, to Kevin Chriss, who showed me that with the right kind of backup, miracles were possible. And special, life-long thanks to Kay Cessna, who knew all too well what I was up against and convinced me not only to begin, but ensured that I had what I needed to finish.

My gratitude to the MacDowell Colony, where I began writing this book, and to the Virginia Center for the Creative Arts, where I finished it. My residencies in those quiet halls provided me with the greatest gift of all—uninterrupted time. A debt of gratitude to the San Francisco Writers' Grotto and all its members—my status as official nomadic office subletter allowed me privacy and space. I look forward to writing the next book in my very own office at the Grotto. And thanks to the Mill Valley Public Library, nestled in a copse of impossibly tall trees, where I thought and wrote, and occasionally stopped to draw a deep breath.

Many authors have had their influence on my thinking, and the ideas that appear in this work emerged from my readings of David Shenk, Steven Johnson, Sharon Begley, Floyd Skloot, Daniel Schacter, Carl Honoré, Denise Grady, Jane Gross, Sandra Blakeslee, Diane Ackerman, Lisa Melton, Will Shortz, James Gleick, Rebecca Rupp, Tara Parker-Pope, Christen Brownlee, Alison Motluck, Gina Kolata, Laurie Tarkan, Natalie Angier, Roni Rabin, Claudia Kalb, Christine Gorman, Jerome Groopman, Ben Harder, Kate Murphy, Ronald Kotulak, Susan Aldridge, Billy Collins, Jared Diamond, Stephanie Saul, Ben Raines and, very much posthumously, Simone de Beauvoir.

It is fortunate that the memory-hungry crowd nervously insists on preserving its anonymity. Otherwise, I'd feel compelled to express my gratitude to every single individual who set aside the hours required to fill out a survey or took the time to meet for a three-hour discussion group. Some people, of course, have gone public: Thus, I can offer my deepest thanks to Lawrence Roberts, Zvi Danenberg, Richard Lang,

Nan Wiener, Dawn Swanson, Courtenay "Co" Crocker and William McGlynn.

It is worth noting, I believe, that in the course of over three years of research, exactly three scientists—out of a group that ultimately exceeded three hundred—turned down a request from me for an interview. Everybody else—whether very eminent or not yet so—simply asked when I wanted to visit or talk over the phone. To a journalist, accustomed to having the door shut in her face and the phone slammed down in her ear, such warm invitations were remarkable. I was impressed, always, by their precision, patience and dedication. Many scientists spent substantial hours with me, patiently explaining their work, grasping that I—like all science reporters who write for a lay audience—would snatch what seemed important, inevitably leaving many of the valuable particulars lying on the laboratory floor. Others in the lab deserve thanks: the small creatures with the long tails. Every time I mention a rodent study, it means that dozens or hundreds of these animals were sacrificed in the pursuit of scientific advancement. You'll never find me wearing so much as a fur-lined glove, but I recognize how crucial these animals are to understanding and curing Alzheimer's, a disease that will otherwise swamp us.

In alphabetical order, I wish to acknowledge the important contributions of the following scientists, physician and mental health professionals: Marilyn Albert, the Alzheimer's Association of America, Karen Ashe, Tallie Baram, Samuel Barondes, George Bartzokis, Gordon Bell, David Bennett, Jan Born, Peter Breggin, Douglas Bremner, Robert Diaz-Brinton, Randy Buckner, Stephen Bunker, Larry Cahill, Jonathan Canick, Anjan Chatterjee, Anthony Chen, Antonio Convit, Carl Cotman, Suzanne Craft, Thomas Crook III, Margaret Cullen, Ward Dean, Mony de Leon, Gayatri Devi, David Dinges, Deborah Dorsey, Richard Doty, Martha Farah, Steven Ferris, Steven Fowkes, Laura Fratiglioni, Bruce Friedman, Richard A. Friedman, Fred Gage, Michaela Gallagher, Joseph Glenmullen, Paul Gold, Elkhonen Goldberg, Elizabeth Gould, Cheryl Grady, Joe Graedon, Robert C. Green, Margaret Gullette, Edward Hallowell, Davis Hasker, Stephen Hauser, Jeff Hawkins, Jane Hightower, James Joseph, Marcel

Just, Eric Kandel, Andrea Kaplan, Lawrence Katz, Claudia Kawas, Dharma Singh Khalsa, Miia Kivipelto, William Klunk, Peter Kramer, Jeffrey Kreutzer, Tracy Kuo, Ray Kurzweil, Margie Lachman, Virginia Lee, Harriet Lerner, Ed Levin, Elizabeth Loftus, Sonia Lupien, Constantine Lyketsos, Kate Mahaffey, Chester Mathis, Mark McDaniel, Bruce McEwen, James McGaugh, Tracy McIntosh, Michael Meaney, Michael Merzenich, David Meyer, Peter Meyers, Karen Miller, John C. Morris, Charles Nemeroff, Maud Nerman, Denise C. Park, Michael Perlis, David Perlmutter, Ronald C. Petersen, Dorene Rentz, Jacqueline Rogers, Benno Roozendaal, Steven P. Rose, Anthony Rostain, Ronald Ruff, Henry Rusinek, Oliver Sacks, Barbara Sahakian, Marvin Sams, Robert Sapolsky, Judith Saxton, Andrew Saykin, Daniel Schacter, Richard Shames, Barbara Sherwin, Daniel Siegel, Gary Small, Scott Small, Susan Smalley, Yaakov Stern, Robert J. Sternberg, Robert Stickgold, Rudolph Tanzi, Pierre Tariot, Harry M. Tracy, John Q. Trojanowski, Tim Tully, Danielle Turner, Mark Tuszynski, Eve Van Cauter, Jeffry Vaught, Joe Verghese, Norma Volkow, Alan Wallace, Michael W. Weiner, Polly Wheat, Aaron White, Robert S. Wilson, Cody Wright, Bruce Yankner and Liqin Zhao.

And finally, with love and from the bottom of my heart, I thank my husband, Ron Ramin, and my sons, Avery and Oliver, for maintaining their conviction that this was a story worth telling, even if it meant that on many days, I forgot far more than I remembered.

RESOURCES

. . .

For a list of thyroid doctors, go to http://thyroid.about.com/cs/doctors/a/topdocs.htm.

For a searchable list of clinical trials, go to http://www.clinicaltrials.gov.

The Alzheimer's Disease Neuroimaging Initiative (ADNI) seeks research participants. For more information, call the Alzheimer's Disease Education and Referral (ADEAR) Center at 1-800-438-4380.

NOTES

· · ·

PREFACE
MOST PRECIOUS POSSESSION
  xv In *The Starr Report*   Daniel Schacter, *The Seven Sins of Memory: How the Mind Forgets and Remembers* (Boston: Houghton Mifflin, 2001), 4–5.

xvii Gary Small . . . phoned   Gary Small, interview by the author, December 1, 2003.

  xx he jogged between eight and fifteen miles a day   Zvi Danenberg, meeting with the author, September 6, 2005.

1. YOUR UNRELIABLE BRAIN
Midlife Forgetfulness Is Embarrassing and Frustrating, but What Does It Mean for the Future?

  3 "normal" . . . defined that word as the dictionary does   *The American Heritage Stedman's Medical Dictionary* (Boston: Houghton Mifflin, 2002).

  5 decaying of memory . . . begins in our twenties   Denise Park, in a paper presented at the American Psychological Association meeting, August 24, 2001.

  5 "It's not the fact of the memory deficit that's the problem"   Harriet Lerner, interview by the author, June 21, 2006.

  7 Alzheimer's occurs in 35 percent of people eighty and older   Gina Kolata, "Live Long, Die Young? Answer Isn't Just in Genes," *New York Times*, August 31, 2006, http://www.nytimes.com.

  7 "Dementia is an ever-deepening advance of wintry whiteness"   George F. Will, "A Mother's Love, Clarified," *Washington Post*, July 13, 2006, A23.

7 I met Phyllis   Phyllis, interview by the author, September 8, 2006.

8 Today, 4.5 million Americans have Alzheimer's   Richard J. Hodes, "Public Funding for Alzheimer Disease Research in the United States," *Nature Medicine*, 12 (July 2006): 770–773.

8 nearly as prevalent in Japan and Europe   Ibid., 778, 774.

9 In 2005, Alzheimer's cost the federal government   Ibid., 780.

9 "By the time even the earliest symptoms of Alzheimer's are detectable"   John C. Morris, interview by the author, July 20, 2004.

9 "If we can meet this disease in the early stage"   John Trojanowski, interview by the author, April 27, 2004.

10 David Bennett, the director of the Alzheimer's Disease Center at Rush   David Bennett, interview by the author, August 7, 2006; David Bennett et al., "Mild Cognitive Impairment Is Related to Alzheimer Disease Pathology and Cerebral Infarctions," *Neurology*, 64 (March 8, 2005): 834–841.

2. GLITCHES, GAPS AND GAFFES
The Memory-Hungry Crowd Speaks Candidly About Screwing Up

17 essay in the *Atlantic Monthly*   Ian Frazier, "If Memory Doesn't Serve," *Atlantic Monthly*, October 2004, 103.

19 men refusing to stop to ask for directions   Daniel Schacter, *The Seven Sins of Memory*, 21.

20 developing software that scans e-mails   "See Attachment (No File Attached)," *New Scientist*, July 29, 2006, 25.

3. FRONTAL-LOBE OVERLOAD
"Too Much Information" Is Just One of the Reasons You Feel Like You're Drowning

24 frontal lobes guide the organization and prioritization   Edward Hallowell, "Overloaded Circuits: Why Smart People Underperform," *Harvard Business Review*, January 1, 2005, 54–61.

25 Homo sapiens traded off a chunk of working memory   "What Only a Chimp Knows," *New Scientist*, June 10, 2006, 48.

25 working memory is "the mental glue"   Daniel Goleman, "Biologists Find Site of Working Memory," *New York Times*, May 2, 1995, C1.

26 neuroscientist Denise Park calls "background noise."   Denise C. Park and Michele L. Meade, "Everyday Memory," in D. Ekerdt, ed., *The MacMillan Encyclopedia of Aging*, 4th ed. (New York: MacMillan Reference, in press).

26 psychiatrist and author Edward M. Hallowell   Edward Hallowell, interview by the author, April 24, 2006.

28 the Blue Man Group   David Shenk, *Data Smog: Surviving the Information Glut* (New York: HarperEdge, 1997), 36.

28 we plug up our ears, pinch our nose Ibid., 102.

29 diagnosis of "neurasthenia" Michelle Stacey, *The Fasting Girl: A True Victorian Medical Mystery* (New York: Tarcher/Penguin, 2002), 9.

29 Vannevar Bush Shenk, *Data Smog*, 62.

30 In his book, *In Praise of Slowness* Carl Honoré, *In Praise of Slowness: How a Worldwide Movement Is Challenging the Cult of Speed* (San Francisco: Harper-SanFrancisco, 2004), 35.

30 Robert Archibald, a historian Robert Archibald, *A Place to Remember: Using History to Build Community* (Walnut Creek, CA: Altamira Press, 1999), 125.

31 Adam Bryant wrote a touching farewell letter to his BlackBerry Adam Bryant, "Feeling All Thumbed Out," *New York Times*, May 28, 2006, 5.

32 *oyayubizoku*, the "thumb tribe." James Gleick, *What Just Happened: A Chronicle from the Information Frontier* (New York: Pantheon, 2002), 283.

32 chief technology officer at Palm Jeff Hawkins, interview by the author, August 26, 2004.

33 "The real challenge of modern life" Edward M. Hallowell, *CrazyBusy: Overstretched, Overbooked, and About to Snap! Strategies for Coping in a World Gone ADD* (New York: Ballantine, 2006), 101.

33 quantify the number of distractions and interruptions Alison Motluk, "Got A Minute?" *New Scientist*, June 24, 2006, 46–49.

33 interruptions take up over two hours Ibid., 48.

34 Using neuroimaging, MIT psychologist Yuhong Jiang et al., "fMRI Provides New Constraints on Theories of the Psychological Refractory Period," *Psychological Science*, 15 (6): 390–396.

34 Studies executed by David E. Meyers Melissa Healy, "We're All Multi-tasking, but What's the Cost?" *Los Angeles Times*, July 19, 2004, F1.

34 "If both tasks require strategic thought" Marcel Just, interview by the author, April 20, 2004.

4. BLOCKING, BLANKING AND BEGGING FOR MERCY
Why Words and Thoughts Flee Without Warning

38 explains that name and word blocking Schacter, *The Seven Sins of Memory*, 51.

38 Schacter observes that the concept of blocking exists Ibid., 72–73.

39 older adults produce more unspecific pronouns Deborah Burke, "Memory and Aging," in Gruneberg & Morris, eds., *Aspects of Memory*, 2d ed. Vol. 1: *The Practical Aspects* (Rutledge, 1992), 126.

39 TOTs (tip of the tongue lapses) William Safire, "On Language. Whosit's Whatchamacallit: The Unexplored World of Tongue-Tippers," *New York Times*, January 9, 2005, sec. 6, 20.

39 To fend off a tip-of-the-tongue incident Daniel Schacter, interview by the author, October 25, 2005.

39 "people can produce virtually everything" Schacter, *The Seven Sins of Memory*, 74.

39 "ugly sisters," unwanted and intrusive words   Schacter, *The Seven Sins of Memory*, 75.

40 turning a concept ... into a word   Susan Kemper and Reinhold Kliegl, eds., *Constraints on Language: Aging, Grammar, and Memory* (Kluwer Academic Publishers, 1999), 89.

40 at the lexeme level, you assemble the components   Burke, "Memory and Aging," 127–128.

41 a nomenclatur, an alert slave   Rebecca Rupp, *Committed to Memory: How We Remember and Why We Forget* (New York: Crown, 1997), 198–199.

41 you should introduce two people, but have blocked on their names   Barbara Wallraff, "Word Fugitives," *Atlantic Monthly*, July/August 2005, 160.

42 Comedian and talk show host Joan Rivers   Bob Morris, "Nice to Meet You ... Again," *New York Times*, December 15, 2002, sec. 9, p. 4.

43 Arthur ... doesn't remember faces   Arthur, interview by the author, November 23, 2004.

44 The lack of facial recognition   Rusiko Bourtchouladze, *Memories Are Made of This: How Memory Works in Humans and Animals* (New York: Columbia University Press, 2002), 60.

5. INTO THE DOUGHNUT HOLE
What a Brain Scan Can (and Cannot) Tell You About
What's Going On Upstairs

45 Gary Small ... author of *The Memory Bible*   Gary Small, *The Memory Bible: An Innovative Strategy for Keeping Your Brain Young* (New York: Hyperion, 2002).

46 I gave him the lowdown on my cognitive state   Gary Small, interview by the author, December 12, 2003.

46 "The metabolic activity of brain cells"   Gary Small, interview by the author, December 19, 2003.

46 "Is the impairment you perceive getting worse?"   Ibid.

47 There are two forms of Alzheimer's disease   Apoorva Mandavilli, "The Amyloid Code," *Nature Medicine*, July 2006, 748.

47 After sixty-five, it afflicts one out of ten   http://www.alz.org/AboutAD/statistics.asp.

47 Alzheimer's actually began in midlife   Alice Dembner, "Tests Will Predict Who Is Developing Alzheimer's and Who Will Benefit Most from Treatment," *Boston Globe*, July 6, 2004.

48 the Mini-Mental State Exam   M. F. Folstein, S. E. Folstein, and P. R. McHugh, "Mini-Mental State: A Practical Method for Grading the State of Patients for the Clinician," *Journal of Psychiatric Research* 12 (1975): 189–198.

48 the MMSE is sensitive only to overt dementia   John C. Morris and D. T. Villareal, "The Diagnosis of Alzheimer's Disease," *Alzheimer's Disease Review* 3 (1998): 142–152; Pauline Spaan et al., "Early Assessment of Dementia: The Contribution of Different Memory Components," *Neuropsychology* 19, no. 5

(2005): 629–640; Janet Duchek et al., "Failure to Control Prepotent Pathways in Early Stage Dementia of the Alzheimer's Type: Evidence from Dichotic Listening," *Neuropsychology* 19, no. 5 (2005): 687–695.

54 The PET scan measured the rate   Andrea Kaplan, e-mail to the author, October 12, 2005.

56 Gary Small told me that the news was great   Gary Small, interview by the author, May 14, 2004.

6. SWALLOW THIS
The Feeding of a Midlife Brain: Essential Fatty Acids, Omega-3s, Vitamins, Supplements and Plenty of Glucose

58 In supplement form, most antioxidants   Lisa Melton, "The Antioxidant Myth," *New Scientist*, August 5, 2006, 40–43.

59 $23 billion a year   Ibid., 40.

59 about $210 million is spent on micronutrients   Pat Rea, interview by the author, January 7, 2004.

59 ginkgo biloba   Stephen S. Hall, "The Quest for a Smart Pill," *Scientific American*, September 2003.

59 Those who spend money on brain boosters   Don Summerfield, interview by the author, January 7, 2005.

59 The ancient Greeks   http://www.paghat.com/rosemary.html.

59 lemon balm on days that were expected to be cognitively demanding   http://www.bbc.co.uk/1/hi/england/2848655.stm, March 14, 2003.

59 Aristotle preferred to apply a compound   Marius d'Assignyr, *The Art of Memory* (New York: AMS Press, 1985).

59 Indian practitioners of Ayurvedic medicine   http://www.raysahelian.com/bacopa.html.

60 Cotman, the director   Three-year study results presented to American Association for the Advancement of Science Conference, Seattle, February 2004.

60 the 14-Day Memory Prescription Program   Deborah Dorsey, interview by the author, December 16, 2003.

62 a couple of bites of a peanut butter sandwich   Paul Gold, "Fluctuations in Glucose Concentration During Behavioral Testing: Dissociations Both Between Brain Areas and Between Brain and Blood," *Neurobiology of Learning and Memory* 75 (2001): 325–337; Paul Gold and Ewan C. McNay, "Age-Related Differences in Hippocampal Extracellular Fluid Glucose Concentration During Behavioral Testing and Following Systemic Glucose Administration," *Journal of Gerontology Series A: Biological Sciences and Medical Sciences* 56 (May 2001): B66–B71.

62 blood levels of glucose influence   Paul Gold, interview by the author, February 16, 2004.

62 Complex carbs   Bijal Trivedi, "The Good, the Fad and the Unhealthy," *New Scientist*, September 23, 2006, 42–48.

63 James Joseph, the director of the neuroscience lab   James Joseph, interview by the author, March 26, 2004.

63 rats that were fed extract of blueberries   J. A. Joseph et al., "Anthocyanins in Aged Blueberry-Fed Rats Are Found Centrally and May Enhance Memory," *Nutritional Neuroscience*, 8, no. 2(April 2005): 111–120; J. A. Joseph et al., "Modulation of Hippocampal Plasticity and Cognitive Behavior by Short-Term Blueberry Supplementation in Aged Rats," *Nutritional Neuroscience* 7, no. 5/6 (2004): 309–316.

63 several fruits and vegetables that adorn themselves in quiet neutrals   "Compound in Apples May Help Fight Alzheimer's disease," American Chemical Society press release, November 16, 2004.

63 Research shows that Indians   "Curry Ingredient May Stop Alzheimer's," Yomiuri Shimbun press release about a paper presented at the Japanese Society of Dementia Research, in Tokyo, September 30, 2004.

64 Peanuts (straight from the shells   Jun Tan et al., "Green Tea Epigallocateden-3-Gallate (EGCG) Modulates Amyloid Precursor Protein Cleavage and Reduces Cerebral Amyloidosis in Alzheimer Transgene Mice." *Journal of Neuroscience*, September 21, 2005, (25) 8807–8814.

64 apples and apple juice   "UMass Lowell Research Shows Benefits of Apple Juice on Neurotransmitter Affecting Memory," University of Massachusetts-Lowell press release, August 1, 2006.

64 omega-3s subdivide into two fatty acids   David Perlmutter, *The Better Brain Book* (New York: Riverhead Books, 2004), 111.

64 EFAs make the membrane more fluid   Trivedi, *New Scientist,* 48.

64 facilitate the production of brain-derived neurotropic factor   Christen Brownlee, "Eat Smart: Foods May Effect the Brain as well as the Body," *Science News*, March 4, 2006, 136.

65 EFAs are so desirable   "This Transgenic Little Piggy Boosts Your Brain," *New Scientist,* April 1, 2006, 20.

65 You'd have to eat five enriched eggs   Alison Motluck, "Aisle Spy: The Hot New Health Foods," *O Magazine*, May 2006, 156.

65 fatty acids . . . a natural curve   Perlmutter, *Better Brain Book*, 26.

65 Trans fats can get in the way   Jane Brody, "Butter or Margarine? First, Study the Label," *New York Times*, September 5, 2006, D7.

66 Brain Sustain   See http://www.inutritionals.com.

66 The magnesium is important   "Magnesium Shown to Boost Learning, Memory," MIT press release, December 2, 2004; "Magnesium May Reverse Middle-Age Memory Loss," MIT press release, December 17, 2004.

67 Andrew Weil answered questions   See http://www.drweil.com.

67 The first time I met Khalsa   Dharma Khalsa Singh, interview by the author, March 15, 2003.

67 antioxidants in supplement   Tara Parker-Pope, "The Case Against Vitamins" *Wall Street Journal*, March 20, 2006, R1.

68 Khalsa beamed at me over a scraggly white beard   Dharma Khalsa Singh, interview by the author, February 20, 2004.

69 B-12 is essential   Perlmutter, *Better Brain Book*, 106.

69 A deficit in B-1   See http://www.whfoods.com/genpage.php?tname=nutrient &dbid=100.

69 Niacin, also a B vitamin   M. C. Morris et al., "Dietary Niacin and the Risk of Incident Alzheimer's Disease and of Cognitive Decline," *Journal of Neurology, Neurosurgery and Psychiatry* 75 (2004): 1093–1099.

69 Folic acid (also known as folate)   "Leafy Green Vegetables May Help Keep Brains Sharp Through Aging," Tufts press release, September 22, 2005.

69 subjects took twice the RDA for folate   "Folic Acid Improves Memory and Protects the Brain from Aging," *Medical Study News*, June 22, 2005.

69 When folic acid combines with B-12   J. Durga et al., "Folate and the Methylene-tetrahydrofolate Reductase 677C-T Mutation Correlate with Cognitive Performance," *Neurobiology of Aging* 27, no. 2 (February 2006): 334–343.

69 Elevated homocysteine   Perlmutter, *Better Brain Book*, 47.

69 consequently diminishing cerebral blood flow   M. A. McDaniels et al., "Brain-Specific Nutrients: A Memory Cure?" *Psychological Science in the Public Interest*, 3 (2002):12–13.

69 High blood levels of homocysteine   Merrill F. Elias, "Homocysteine and Cognitive Performance in the Framingham Offspring Study: Age Is Important," *American Journal of Epidemiology* 162, no. 7 (2005): 644–653.

69 1,000 IUs of vitamin C and 1,000 IUs of vitamin E   Peter Zandi, "Reduced Risk of Alzheimer's Disease in Users of Antioxidant Vitamin Supplements," *Archives of Neurology*, no. 61 (January 2004): 82–88.

69 results showing that large doses of vitamin E   "Effects of Long-term Vitamin E Supplementation on Cardiovascular Events and Cancer: A Randomized Controlled Trial," *Journal of the American Medical Association* 293, no. 11 (2005): 1338–1347.

70 Although evidence for gingko's effectiveness is marginal   Peter A. G. M. DeSmet, "$283 Million Reimbursed by German Health Insurance," *New England Journal of Medicine* 352 (March 24, 2005): 1176–1178.

70 Current thinking on gingko   P. R. Solomon et al., "Ginkgo for Memory Enhancement: A Randomized Controlled Trial," *Journal of the American Medical Association* 288, no. 7 (2002): 835–840.

70 phosphytidyl serine, known as PS   McDaniels, "Brain-Specific Nutrients."

70 The amino acid called acetyl-L-carnitine   Ibid.

70 There was also vinpocetine   Ibid.

7. MENTAL AEROBICS
From Tedious to Addictive: Options for Exercising Your Neurons

73 I'd had such little success with mental aerobics   Deborah Dorsey, interview by the author, January 27, 2004.

75 ordinary people can use imagery mnemonics   Daniel Schacter, *The Seven Sins of Memory*, 34.

75 skepticism about the value of mnemonics Lawrence Katz, interview by the author, April 22, 2004.

76 try approaching your front door with your eyes closed Lawrence Katz, *Keep Your Brain Alive—83 Neurobic Exercises* (New York: Workman, 1998).

77 "The world is really the best brain gym" Katz interview.

77 "When you're packing up your stuff for the day" Ibid.

78 developed a program called HiFi Michael Merzenich, interview by the author, April 20, 2005.

78 The brain has about 100 billion neurons Nicholas Wade, "Brains and Brawn: One and the Same," *New York Times*, January 25, 2004, D7.

78 Plasticity reflects the brain's ability to reorganize itself Randy Buckner, interview by the author, September 12, 2005.

78 Clusters of neurons Merzenich interview.

78 The existing troops are continuously reinforced Ibid.

79 Increased mental and physical exercise Ibid.

79 "Here's why you lose your memory in midlife" Ibid.

79 hearing loss is often a factor in . . . forgetfulness Arthur Wingfield et al., "Hearing Loss in Older Adulthood: What It Is and How It Interacts with Cognitive Performance," *Current Directions in Psychological Science* 14, no. 3 (2005): 144–148.

79 The software costs $495 Kerry A. Dolan, "Sharp as a Tack," *Forbes*, March 27, 2006.

80 chief scientific officer of Posit Science Merzenich interview.

80 audio form of Concentration Merzenich interview.

81 determined to attract not only boomers, but members of Gen X Bruce Friedman, interview by the author, February 12, 2006.

82 "I had the sense that my mind was slowing down" Bill McGlynn, e-mail to the author, February 13, 2006.

83 he takes on the MBT Challenge Ibid.

83 Brain Age Walter S. Mossberg, "Survived the '60s? You May Want to Try This Nintendo Game," *Wall Street Journal*, March 23, 2006. Viewed at http://ptech.wsj.com/archive/ptech-20060323.html.

8. BATHING IN BATTERY ACID
Elevated Cortisol Associated with Chronic Stress Is No Friend to Your Hippocampus

85 "Sometimes I pay the closest attention possible" Jeanette, interview by the author, April 19, 2004.

85 It is a framer, a setter-in-context Bruce McEwen, *The End of Stress As We Know It* (Washington, DC: National Academies Press, 2002), 62.

86 An occasional burst of stress can be neuroprotective Lyle E. Bourne Jr. and Rita A. Yaroush, "Stress and Cognition: A Cognitive Psychological Perspective," *National Aeronautics and Space Administration*, February 1, 2003, 23ff.

86 To meet the scientific definition of stress Sonia Lupien, "New Research Stresses the Responses to Stress," *BrainWork*, March/April 2004, 1.

86 " ... about three minutes of screaming terror" Robert Sapolsky, *Monkeyluv and Other Essays on Our Lives as Animals* (New York: Scribner, 2005), 101.

86 "The human mind is so powerful" Bruce McEwen, interview by the author, December 7, 2005.

87 Even a few days of elevated cortisol Ibid.

87 (Other hormones in the body decline Robert Sapolsky, *Why Zebras Don't Get Ulcers: A Guide to Stress, Stress-Related Diseases, and Coping* (New York: W. H. Freeman, 1994).

87 three weeks of repeated stress McEwen, *End of Stress*, 123.

88 chronically high levels of cortisol Robert Sapolsky, "Taming Stress," *Scientific American*, September 2003, 92.

88 once the stress response is shut down McEwen interview.

89 The cycle starts with elevated cortisol McEwen, *End of Stress*, 122–123.

89 depression is sixty times rarer Trivedi, *New Scientist*, 48.

89 hippocampal injury accumulates with recurrent depressive episodes Sapolsky, "Taming Stress."

90 "SSRIs require about a month" Fred Gage, "Depression and the Birth and Death of Brain Cells," *American Scientist* 88, no. 4 (2000): 340.

90 Post-traumatic stress disorder R. C. Kessler et al., "Posttraumatic Stress Disorder in the National Comorbidity Survey," *Archives of General Psychiatry* 52, no 12 (1995):1048–1060.

90 "Post-traumatic stress disorder patients have their fear alarms" Douglas Bremner, *Does Stress Damage the Brain? Understanding Trauma-Related Disorders from a Mind-Body Perspective* (New York: Norton, 2002), 152.

90 In a neuropsychological study of patients with PTSD Douglas Bremner, interview by the author, June 1, 2004.

91 "Stress proneness" Robert Wilson, "Proneness to Psychological Distress Is Associated with Risk of Alzheimer's Disease," *Neurology* 61 (2003): 1479–1485.

91 stressed or depressed mothers and their unborn babies Laurie Tarkan, "Tracking Stress and Depression Back to the Womb," *New York Times*, December 7, 2004, D5.

92 infants placed in unfamiliar environments "New Research Stresses the Responses to Stress," *Brainwork*, March/April 2004, 3.

92 the relationship of rat pups and their mothers "Early Life Psychological Stress Can Lead to Memory Loss and Cognitive Decline in Middle Age," *Journal of Neuroscience*, University of California-Irvine press release, October 12, 2005.

92 The problem, Baram found, emerged from deep in the brain Ibid.

94 In his "licking behavior" rat study Brenda Patoine, "Parenting Matters: Your Genes Prove It," *BrainWork: The Neuroscience Newsletter*, January-February 2005, 8.

94 The more care a pup received Ibid.

94 rats and humans share about 90 percent Ben Karpf, "New Rat Genome Se-

quence Could Offer Benefits, Researchers Say," *U.S. Medicine*, May 2004. Viewed at http://www.usmedicine.com/article.cfm?articleID=867&issueID=62.

96 when mothers are emotionally unavailable   Daniel Siegel, *The Developing Mind: Toward a Neurobiology of Interpersonal Experience* (New York: Guilford Press, 1999), 119–120.

96 I telephoned Siegel   Daniel Siegel, interview by the author, May 5, 2005.

9. YEARNING FOR ESTROGEN
Rejecting Hormone Therapy Could Leave Your Neurons in the Lurch

99 Sufficient levels of the hormone are essential   Bruce McEwen, *The End of Stress As We Know It*, 168–169.

99 Estrogen also increases the rate of neurogenesis   Pauline Maki, "Estrogen Effects on the Hippocampus and Frontal Lobes," *International Journal of Fertility and Women's Medicine* 50, no. 2 (2005): 67–71.

99 The hormone has shown a remarkable ability   C. Kawas et al., "Treating Alzheimer's Disease: Today and Tomorrow," *Patient Care*, November 15, 1996, 62–83.

99 Estrogen also helps protect brain cells   Bruce C. McEwen and Stephen E. Alves, "Estrogen Actions in the Central Nervous System," *Endocrine Reviews* 20, no. 3 (1999): 279–307.

99 [Estrogen] stimulat[es] glucose metabolism   Maki, "Estrogen Effects."

99 it may also slow the shrinkage of gray matter   K. I. Erickson et al., "Selective Sparing of Brain Tissue in Postmenopausal Women Receiving Hormone Replacement Therapy," *Neurobiology of Aging* 26, no. 8 (2005): 1205–1213.

99 one-third of her life in postmenopause   Natalie Rasgon, ed., *The Effects of Estrogen on Brain Function* (Baltimore, MD: Johns Hopkins University Press, 2006), 1.

99 "estrogen is critical"   Robert Sapolsky, interview by the author, November 18, 2005.

99 The difference in tests of verbal fluency   Dr. Barbara Sherwin, e-mail correspondence, June 13, 2004.

99 Women's Health Initiative   "Ob/Gyn Panel Revisits HRT," Yale University press release, October 29, 2004.

99 hormone therapy . . . could prevent coronary heart disease   Rasgon, *Effects of Estrogen.*

100 the WHI produced nothing but bad news   Roni Rabin, "Basing Choice on Risk vs. Benefit," *New York Times*, January 31, 2006.

100 If HRT was prescribed at all   American College of Obstetricians and Gynecologists, "Frequently Asked Questions About Hormone Therapy." Viewed at http://www.acog.org (October 2004).

101 tried to wean herself off HRT   Jane Gross, "Strokes or Insomnia? A Woman's Hormone Quandary," *New York Times*, March 23, 2004, D5.

102 Gayatri Devi . . . runs the New York Memory Clinic   Gayatri Devi, interview by the author, June 8, 2004.

103 "The kinds of skills required of a middle-aged woman at home" Ibid.

103 specific types of memory remained perfectly intact Peter Meyers, "A Population-Based Longitudinal Study of Cognitive Functioning in the Menopausal Transition," *Neurology* 61(2003): 801–806.

103 twenty-four perimenopausal women "Memory Problems at Menopause: Nothing to Forget About," University of Rochester press release, February 3, 2006.

103 "I've known that researchers were giving the wrong tests" Devi interview.

104 An ancillary trial called WHIMS Ingrid Wickelgren, "Brain Researchers Try to Salvage Estrogen Treatments," *Science* 302 (2003): 1138–1139.

105 At the start of the [WHI] study Barbara Sherwin, "Surgical Menopause, Estrogen, and Cognitive Function in Women: What Do the Findings Tell Us?" *Annals of the New York Academy of Science* 1052 (2005): 3–10.

105 "window of opportunity" Ibid.

105 Prempro . . . can be sedating Rasgon, *Effects of Estrogen on Brain Function*, 31–32.

105 women who used both progesterone and estrogen Ibid., 33.

106 balanced with progesterone Sherwin, "Surgical Menopause," 5.

106 promoting cognitive function Rasgon, *Effects of Estrogen on Brain Function*, 127.

106 Brinton's lab has produced 32 molecules Ibid., 132.

106 "a neuroSERM would have to behave as an estrogen" Liqin Zhao, "Estrogen Receptor β as a Therapeutic Target for Promoting Neurogenesis and Preventing Neurodegeneration," in press.

106 Because neuroSERMs lack the feminizing effects Liqin Zhao et al., "Selective Estrogen Receptor Modulators (SERMs) for the Brain: Current Status and Remaining Challenges for Developing NeuroSERMs," *Brain Research Reviews* 49 (2005): 472–493.

107 closely linked to the level of estrogen present in the brain Roberta Diaz Brinton, "Impact of Estrogen Therapy on Alzheimer's Disease: A Fork in the Road?" *CNS Drugs* 18 (2004): 405–422.

107 women who died with Alzheimer's Rena Li et al., "Brain Estrogen Deficiency Accelerates Abeta Plaque Formation in an Alzheimer's Disease Animal Model," *Proceedings of the National Academy of Sciences* 102, no. 52 (2005): 19198–19203.

107 Men who develop Alzheimer's "Androgen Loss May Lead to Alzheimer's," University of Southern California press release, September 21, 2004.

107 black cohosh "Sleight of Herb: Black Cohosh Mislabeled in Medicinal Products," *Science News*, May 13, 2006, 293.

107 In the wake of the WHI study Claudia Kalb, "How to Lift the Mind: For Those Suffering from the Pain of Anxiety and Depression, Complementary Medicine Is No Miracle Cure. But Some Treatments Offer Real Hope," *Newsweek*, December 2, 2002.

108 Data from the Nurses' Health Study Rabin, "Basing Choice on Risk vs. Benefit."

10. THE VULNERABLE BRAIN
The Repercussions of Concussions You Never Knew You Had

109 I called Gary Small to ask   Gary Small, interview by the author, May 14, 2004.

110 Jonathan Canick phoned   Jonathan Canick, interview by the author, November 24, 2003.

111 an appointment to go see   Jonathan Canick, interview by the author, December 4, 2003.

114 diffusion tensor imaging   "New Brain Imaging Reveals Damage MRI Misses," *Good Morning America*, February 17, 2006; viewed at http:www.abcnews.go.com/GMA/story?1d=1627855&page=1; N. Nakayama, "Evidence for White Matter Disruption in Traumatic Brain Injury Without Microscopic Lesions," *Journal of Neurology, Neurosurgery, and Psychiatry* 77, no. 7 (2006): 850–855.

114 can trace axon fiber tracts in the brain   Gary Abrams, e-mail to the author, November 23, 2004.

114 a mild traumatic brain injury result in cognitive deficits   D. H. Smith et al., "Accumulation of Amyloid [beta] and Tau and the Formation of Neurofilament Inclusions Following Diffuse Brain Injury in the Pig," *Journal of Neuropathology and Experimental Neurology* 58 (1999): 982–992, as reported in the Franklin Institute Online, http://www.fi.edu/brain/head.htm.

114 It also stepped up the formation of amyloid plaques   "New Study at UNC Shows Concussions Promote Dementias in Retired Professional Football Players," University of North Carolina press release, October 10, 2005.

116 at least 1.1 million people each year sustain MTBIs   National Center for Injury Prevention and Control, "Report to Congress on Mild Traumatic Brain Injury in the United States: Steps to Prevent a Serious Public Health Problem," Centers for Disease Control and Prevention, September 2003, as reported in "Incidence of Mild and Moderate Brain Injury in the United States, 1991," *Brain Injury* 10, no. 1 (1996): 47–54.

120 Sports injuries account for more than 20 percent   Ibid.

120 one high school football player in five suffers a concussion   Jane Brody, "In Sports, Play Smart and Watch Your Head," *New York Times*, October 26, 2004, F9.

120 The subtle effects of a concussion   "NFL Players Show More Rapid Recovery from Concussions than High School Players," University of Pittsburgh Medical Center press release, January 23, 2006.

121 A computerized battery of neurocognitive tests called IMPACT   Ibid.

121 drugs used to treat the early stages of Alzheimer's   "The Johns Hopkins White Paper Bulletins," *Memory*, April 22, 2005, 11.

121 track cellular debris   John Pastor, "Biomarker Test May Give Early Warning of Brain Woes," University of Florida News, October 13, 2005.

11. COSMETIC NEUROLOGY
The Potential for Pharmaceutical Cognitive Enhancement
Is Vast and Possibly Irresistible

124 people with specific frontal-lobe deficits in attention   Anthony Rostain, interview by the author, October 3, 2004.

124 amphetamines, which the FDA has included in its list of Schedule II drugs   Controlled Substances Act definition, http://www.dea.gov/pubs/csa/801.htm.

124 1.7 million adults ages twenty to sixty-four and 3.3 million children   "ADHD Drug Use in US Rose Among Ages 20 to 44," Medco Health Solutions press release, March 21, 2006.

125 ARPANET, the military technology that led to the invention of the Internet   Lawrence Roberts, interview by the author, August 16, 2004.

125 Jean-Paul Sartre . . . took stimulants every day   John Lanchester, "High Style: Writing Under the Influence," *The New Yorker*, January 6, 2003.

126 10 milligrams, about the same quantity that a pediatrician would prescribe   *Physician's Desk Reference*, 58th edition (New Jersey: Thomson PDR, 2003).

129 the drugs were potentially more dangerous to the heart   Gardiner Harris, "Warning Urged on Stimulants Like Ritalin," *New York Times*, February 10, 2006.

129 the FDA had approved Provigil   Michael Perlis, interview by the author, March 4, 2005.

129 Provigil for the treatment of excessive daytime sleepiness   Viewed at http://www.cephalon.com.

130 unlike Adderall and other psychostimulants   Jerome Groopman, "Eyes Wide Open," *The New Yorker*, December 3, 2001.

130 exactly how Provigil enhanced alertness   Jeffrey Vaught, interview by the author, February 8, 2006.

130 Provigil isn't very different from drinking coffee   Ibid.

130 modafinil (the generic name for Provigil)   Graham Lawton, "The New Incredibles: Enhanced Humans," *New Scientist*, May 13, 2006; Danielle C. Turner et al., "Cognitive Enhancing Effects of Modafinil in Healthy Volunteers," *Psychopharmacology* 165 (2003): 260–269.

131 "People are more reflective"   Danielle Turner, interview by the author, February 2, 2006.

131 Anthony Chen, M.D., a research fellow in cognitive neuroscience   Anthony Chen, interview by the author, November 15, 2004.

134 sales of Provigil climbed 51 percent   "Cephalon Breaks $1B in Revenue," *Philadelphia Business Journal*, February 15, 2005.

134 Adderall, with sales of $1.16 billion in 2005   Anna Wilde Mathews and Scott Hensley, "Strong ADHD Drug Alerts Are Urged: FDA Might Not Heed Advice of Split Advisory Committee About Heart-Risk Labeling," *Wall Street Journal*, February 10, 2006.

135 it would be remembered not as a drug for the treatment of narcolepsy   Turner interview.

135 Provigil for ADHD   "ADHD Drug Snag," *New Scientist*, August 19, 2006, 7.

135 There are about forty cognition-enhancing drugs   "The New Incredibles," *New Scientist*.

136 the company that develops a drug to safely improve cognition   Harry M. Tracy, "Mild Cognitive Impairment," *Neuroinvestment* 102, November 2003; "Memory Deficits," *Neuroinvestment* 126, November 2005.

136 The goal is to discover drug compounds that can modulate memory   Catherine Arnst, "I Can't Remember: Drugs to Stave Off Memory Impairment May Be on the Horizon," *BusinessWeek*, September 1, 2003.

136 "protect and enhance the function of the human mind"   Viewed at http://www.saegispharma.com.

136 approval for treatment of more serious disorders   *Neuroinvestment* 102, November 2003.

136 the agency is mistakenly operating under the assumption   Harry Tracy, interview by the author, July 29, 2004.

137 elevated levels of BDNF   E. Jaffe, "Total Recall: Drug Shows Long-Lasting Boosts of Memory in Rats," *New Scientist*, August 12, 2006, 101.

137 problems lie in deficits of attention and working memory   A. F. T. Arnsten et al., "Dysregulation of Protein Kinase A Signaling in the Aged Prefrontal Cortex: New Strategy for Treating Age-Related Cognitive Decline," *Neuron* 40 (2003): 835–845.

137 Eric Wasserman, who is head of the brain stimulation unit   Bijal Trivedi, "Electrify Your Mind—Literally," *New Scientist*, April 15, 2006.

137 "like giving a cup of coffee to a relatively focal part of the brain"   Ibid., 36.

137 It's a tiny current, between one and two milliamps   Ibid., 34.

137 Francis Fukuyama, author of *Our Posthuman Future*   Ronald Bailey, "The Battle for Your Brain," Reasononline, February 2003, http://www.reason.com/0302/fe.rb.the.shtml.

138 "safe and effective method of enhancing memory,"   Martha Farah, interview by the author, April 26, 2004.

138 working memory and total recall   "As Evolution Intended," *New Scientist*, August 26, 2006, 25.

12. MEDITATION AND NEUROFEEDBACK
Going Iin for a Tune-up: Why Tinkering with Brain Waves Can Improve Attention

139 In mindfulness, instead of struggling to suppress thoughts   Scott R. Bishop et al., "Mindfulness: A Proposed Operational Definition," *Clinical Psychology: Science and Practice* II, no. 3, 230–241, September 2004.

139 the training taught you how to sustain attention   John Teasdale et al., "Mindfulness Training and Problem Formulation," *Clinical Psychology: Science and Practice* 10 (2003):157–160.

140 recommended Margaret Cullen, a clinical psychologist   Alan Wallace, interview by the author, December 7, 2004.

141 Jon Kabat-Zinn developed the first mindfulness-based stress-reduction program   Jon Kabat-Zinn, *Full Catastrophe Living: Using the Wisdom of Your Body and Mind to Face Stress, Pain, and Illness* (New York: Delacorte Press, 1990).

143 I learned about Susan Smalley's efforts   Wallace interview.

143 Mindful Awareness Research Center (MARC) at UCLA   Susan Smalley, interview by the author, February 13, 2006.

143 The training worked   Ibid.

143 MARC Web site   See http://www.marc.ucla.edu.

144 neurofeedback ... could be very expensive and time-consuming   See http://www.bcia.org.

145 When [Sams and I] spoke on the phone   Marvin Sams, interview by the author, December 9, 2004.

145 "We're dealing with the brain"   Ibid.

146 just enough time to clear Provigil from my system   Marvin Sams, interview by the author, January 4, 2005.

148 An experienced Tetris player racks up at least twenty-five thousand points in a game   Marvin Sams, interview by the author, December 9, 2004.

150 Every little bit helped, I told Sams   Marvin Sams, interview by the author, January 24, 2005.

13. I'LL SLEEP WHEN I'M DEAD
Sacrifice Your Slumber and You'll Perform as Well as if
You've Had a Few Stiff Drinks

151 [sleep] declines by twenty-seven minutes each decade   *Journal of the American Medical Association*, August 16, 2000, as cited in "Sleep Linked to Ageing," *BBC News,* August 15, 2000.

151 About forty-two million sleeping pill prescriptions   Stephanie Saul, "Record Sales of Sleeping Pills Are Causing Worries," *New York Times*, February 7, 2006.

151 prescriptions for sleeping pills   Ben Harder, "Staring into the Dark," *Science News*, November 26, 2005.

152 hours of sleep decline in midlife   A. Vgontzas et al., "Middle-Aged Men Show Greater Sensitivity of Sleep to the Arousing Effects of Corticotropin-Releasing Hormone Than Young Men: Clinical Implications," *Journal of Clinical Endocrinology and Metabolism*, 86, no. 4 (2001): 1489–1495.

152 "One complete night of sleep deprivation"   "The Human Brain: The Effects of Sleep Deprivation," Franklin Institute Online, viewed at http://www.fi.edu/brain/sleep.htm.

152 The average adult now sleeps 6.9 hours   2002 "Sleep in America" poll, National Sleep Foundation, March 2002, prepared by WB and A Market, Research Washington, DC.

153 two-thirds of the subjects reported that sleepiness interfered   Ibid.

153 Daytime sleepiness is so common that people take it for granted   Christine Gorman, "Why We Sleep," *Time Magazine*, December 20, 2004.

153 catching a quick nap Dana Sullivan, "How to Nap," *Real Simple*, December 2005-January 2006, 215–218.

153 sleep deprivation . . . activates the hotline to the HPA axis Eve Van Cauter et al., "Age-Related Changes in Slow-Wave Sleep and REM Sleep and Relationship with Growth Hormone and Cortisol Levels in Healthy Men," *Journal of the American Medical Association* 284 (2000): 861–868.

154 say that they experience symptoms of insomnia Jerome Groopman, "Eyes Wide Open," *The New Yorker*, December 3, 2001.

154 "corner of the brain dedicated to niggling anxieties" Robert Stickgold, interview by the author, March 8, 2004.

154 non-REM, followed by REM Ibid.

155 Slow-wave sleep gives the brain Ibid.

155 slow-wave sleep . . . diminishes to just over 3 percent of your sleep in middle age Eve Van Cauter et al., "Age-Related Changes."

155 next-generation sleeping pills "APD125 for Insomnia: Phase 1 Results Provided Evidence of Safety, Increased Time in Slow Wave Sleep, and a Positive Signal on Sleep Maintenance Parameters," Arena Pharmaceuticals, viewed at http://www.arenapharm.com/wt/page/adp125.

156 REM is the cleanup crew Gorman, "Why We Sleep."

156 a plague of insomnia strikes the Colombian village of Macondo Gabriel García Márquez, *One Hundred Years of Solitude* (New York: Harper & Row, 1970).

158 Tracy Kuo, a psychologist at the Stanford University Sleep Disorder Center Tracy Kuo, interview by the author, March 30, 2005.

158 The idea behind CBT is quite simple Michael Perlis, interview by the author, March 4, 2005.

159 One study of CBT-I programs Ibid.

159 I interviewed one of her CBT-I patients Maureen, interview by the author, March 30, 2005.

163 Kuo looked over my sleep diary at my third visit Tracy Kuo, interview by the author, March 23, 2006.

163 obstructive sleep apnea Medline Plus, http://www.nlm.nih.gov/medlineplus/ency/article/000811.htm.

163 obstructive sleep apnea patients are overweight Kuo interview.

164 the struggle for air was waking them up Polo-Kantola, "Sex Steroids and Sleep: Sleep Disturbances in Menopause," *Annals of Endocrinology* 64, no. 2 (2003):152–156.

14. RECREATIONAL DRUGS, ALCOHOL AND OTHER NEUROTOXINS
The Cognitive Consequences of What You Smoke, Drink, Eat and Breathe

166 long-term marijuana users, who smoked four or more joints a week Lambros Messinis et al., "Neuropsychological Deficits in Long-Term Frequent Cannabis Users," *Neurology* 66 (2006): 737–739.

166 Heavy marijuana users experience reduced blood flow Ronald Herning and

Jean Lud Cadet, "Cerebrovascular Perfusion in Marijuana Users During a Month of Monitored Abstinence," *Neurology* 64 (2005): 488–693, February 8, 2005.

166 A healthy hippocampus is studded with acetylcholine receptors   A. J. Gruber et al., "Attributes of Long-Term Heavy Cannabis Users: A Case-Control Study," *Psychological Medicine* 33, no. 8 (2003):1415–1422.

166 MDMA, a synthetic union of psychedelics and amphetamines   Drake Bennett, "Dr. Ecstasy," *New York Times Magazine*, January 30, 2005.

166 cause irreversible damage to the central nervous system   Alison Motluk, "Ecstasy May Damage the Brain's Physical Defenses," *New Scientist*, November 14, 2005.

167 those who had used Ecstasy at least ten times   "Patterns of Drug Use and the Influence of Gender on Self-Reports of Memory Ability in Ecstasy Users: A Web-Based Study," *Journal of Psychopharmacology* 17, no. 4 (2003): 389–396.

167 alcohol can lower your risk for heart attack   Tara Parker-Pope, "Drink Your Medicine? Weighing the Health Benefits, Risks of Alcohol," *Wall Street Journal*, December 28, 2004, D1.

167 alcoholic blackouts   Aaron White, interview by the author, April 22, 2004.

168 "alcohol basically shuts these cells off"   Ibid.

168 continuous consumption of alcohol for as little as eight weeks   Susan A. Farr et al., "Chronic Ethanol Consumption Impairs Learning and Memory After Cessation of Ethanol," *Alcoholism: Clinical and Experimental Research* 29, June 2005: 971–982.

168 "'cocktail party deficits.'"   White interview.

168 alcohol's effect on GABA neural receptors   Richard Olsen et al., "Alcohol-induced Motor Impairment Caused by Increased Extrasynaptic GABA-A Receptor Activity," *Nature Neuroscience* 8: 339–345, February 6, 2005 online edition.

169 The brains of alcoholics are smaller   "Neuroimaging Confirms the Greater Vulnerability of Women's Brains to Alcohol," *Science Daily* press release, May 31, 2005, citing Karl Mann's research in *Alcoholism: Clinical & Experimental Research*, May 2005.

169 during intoxication, neurogenesis . . . stops in its tracks   Kimberly Nixon and Fulton Crews, "Binge Ethanol Exposure Decreases Neurogenesis in Adult Rat Hippocampus," *Journal of Neurochemistry* 83, no. 5 (2002):1087–1093.

169 chronic alcohol abuse alters the expression   Clive Harper et al., "Expression of MBP, PLP, MAG, CNP, and GFAP in the Human Alcoholic Brain," *Alcoholism: Clinical Experimental Research* 29, no. 9 (2005):1698–1705.

169 If heavy drinkers also smoke cigarettes   Beeri M. Schnaider et al., "Diabetes Mellitus in Midlife and the Risk of Dementia Three Decades Later," *Neurology* 63, no. 10 (2004): 1902–1907.

169 People who smoke in midlife   Rachel Whitmer et al., "Midlife Cardiovascular Risk Factors and Risk of Dementia in Late Life," *Neurology* 64 (2005): 277–281.

169 current smokers performed significantly worse   Lawrence Whalley et al.,

"Smoking and Cognitive Change from Age 11 to 66 Years: A Confirmatory Investigation," *Addictive Behaviors*, in press.

170 Methylmercury does its dirty work Jane Hightower, interview by the author, November 10, 2004; "New Study Finds Upper-Income Fish Eaters Exposed to Dangerous Levels of Mercury," National Institute of Environmental Health press release, October 22, 2002. Viewed online at http://www.ehponline.org/press/mercury.html.

170 mercury toxicity "Mercury White Paper," www.epa.gov/oar/whtpaper.pdf; "Mercury and Fish Consuption: Medical and Public Health Issues," 2004 American Medical Association, www.ama-assn.org.ama/pub/category/13619.

170 "Mercury does not belong in the human body" Hightower interview.

170 accident with organic mercury Ibid.

171 the case of Will Smith Ben Raines, "Your Deadly Diet," *Health*, June 2003, 121–122.

171 issued a joint consumer advisory about mercury "What You Need to Know About Mercury in Fish and Shellfish," FDA/EPA Consumer Advisory, March 2004.

172 *all* Americans eat seafood twice a week. "Americans Advised to Eat Seafood Twice a Week," Reuters Health press release, December 21, 2005.

172 The EPA has a "reference dose" Kathryn R. Mahaffey et al., "Blood Mercury Levels in U.S. Children and Women of Childbearing Age 1999–2000," *Journal of the American Medical Association* 289 (April 2003): 1667–1674.

172 mercury levels in salmon Jeffery A. Foran et al., "Quantitative Analysis of the Benefits and Risks of Consuming Farmed and Wild Salmon," *Journal of Nutrition* 135 (November 2005): 2639–2643.

172 California sushi restaurants Jerry Hirsch, "Toxic Tuna in Los Angeles Sushi," *Los Angeles Times*, March 6, 2006. http:www.tunafacts.com/mediacenter/2006_releases/6_06_06_2.html.

172 one billon pounds of canned and "pouched" tuna Trevor Francis's response to *Consumer Reports* story on tuna, U.S. Tuna Foundation, June 6, 2006.

172 personally tested ten cans of tuna for mercury Raines, *Health*, 184.

173 fish guy at Whole Foods Jerry Hirsch, "A Hook for Landing Mercury-Wary Eaters," *Los Angeles Times*, February 27, 2006, www.safeharborfoods.com.

173 Testers extract a sample "How We Test Fish," Safe Harbor Foods 2006, www.safeharborfoods.com/howtest.html.

173 Carbon monoxide poisoning Mona Hopkins, "Gas Attack: Carbon Monoxide Poisoning," Memory Loss and the Brain, Summer 2002, http://www.memorylossonline.com/gasattack.htm.

175 organophosphates reach toxic levels Ed Levin, interview by the author, April 22, 2004.

175 sensitivity to chemical agents Clement E. Furlong, "PON1 Status of Farmworkers, Mothers and Children as a Predictor of Organophosphate Sensitivity," *Pharmacogenetics and Genomics* 16(3):183–190, March 2, 2006.

15. WHAT YOUR DOCTOR FORGOT TO TELL YOU
Prescription Drugs and "Safe" Over-the-Counter Meds May Account for Your Fogginess

177 the FDA does not require   Joe Graedon, interview by the author, May 5, 2003.

180 diphenhydramine caused more driving impairment   John M. Weiler, "Effects of Fexofenadine, Diphenhydramine and Alcohol on Driving Performance," *Annals of Internal Medicine* 132, no. 5 (2000): 354–363.

181 14 percent of Zyrtec users experienced drowsiness   See Pfizer's product labeling for Zyrtec, at http://www.zyrtec.com/.

181 allergic rhinitis   M. S. Blaiss, "Social, Cognitive, and Economic Allergic Rhinitis," *Allergy Asthma Proceedings* 21 (2000): 7–13.

181 studies that demonstrate cortisone's amnesiac effects   P. A. Keenan, "The Effect on Memory of Chronic Prednisone Treatment in Patients with Systemic Disease," *Neurology* 47, no. 6 (1996): 1396–1402, http://www.neurology.org/cgi/content/abstract/47/6/1396.

182 the chemo-treated brain look twenty-five years older than it actually was   Tara Parker-Pope, "Chemo Patients' Memory Loss Is Real, Studies Reveal," *Wall Street Journal*, April 6, 2004, D1.

182 studies of breast-cancer patients   Ibid.

182 neurotoxic effects of chemotherapy   A. F. Saykin, "Neuropsychological Impact of Standard-Dose Systemic Chemotherapy in Long-Term Survivors of Breast Cancer Lymphoma," *Journal of Clinical Oncology* 20, no. 2 (2002): 485–493, http://www.jco.org/cgi/content/abstract/20/2/485.

183 By 1979, one in five women and one in ten men were on benzos   "Use and Abuse of Benzodiazepines," U.S. Government Printing Office, Transcript of a Hearing before the Subcommittee on Health and Scientific Research of the Committee on Labor and Human Resources, Washington, DC: 1980.

183 benzos, which work by enhancing the action of the inhibitory neurotransmitter GABA   Peter Breggin, "Analysis of Adverse Behavioral Effects," *Journal of Mind and Behavior* 19 (Winter 1998): 21–50.

184 "Their primary clinical effect is to induce sedation"   Richard Friedman, interview by the author, December 28, 2004.

184 The drugs are vastly over-prescribed   Ibid.

184 John Irving stopped taking the drugs   Dinitia Smith, "While Excavating Past, Writer Finds His Family," *New York Times*, June 28, 2005, E1.

184 patients complain that they feel blunted on the drugs. Charles Nemeroff, interview by the author, May 31, 2005.

184 scientists suspect that serotonin-based antidepressants   Joseph Glenmullen, interview by the author, September 10, 2005.

184 a specific receptor for dopamine   Nora D. Volkow et al., "Association Between Age-Related Decline in Brain Dopamine Activity and Impairment in Frontal and Cingulate Metabolism," *American Journal of Psychiatry* 157 (January 2000): 75–80.

185 The brain is a highly integrated organ   Peter Breggin and David Cohen, *Your Drug May Be Your Problem: How and Why to Stop Taking Psychiatric Medications* (New York: Perseus, 1999), 36.

185 non-benzo hypnotics . . . can help. Ben Harder, "Staring into the Dark," *Science News*, November 26, 2005.

185 non-benzo hypnotics do not affect sleep architecture   Michael Perlis, interview by the author, March 4, 2005.

185 "You look at the polysomnography"   Ibid.

186 Ambien prescription   Packaging insert.

186 people who have had zombie-type experiences on Ambien   See http://www.websciences.org; and http://www.sleephomepages.org/discussions/basic/messages/msg08802.html.

187 new generation of sleep-enhancing pharmaceuticals   "APD125 for Insomnia: Phase 1 Results Provided Evidence of Safety, Increased Time in Slow Wave Sleep, and a Positive Signal on Sleep Maintenance Parameters," Arena Pharmaceuticals, http://www.arenapharm.com/wt/page/apd125.

187 Lunesta, the longer-acting sleep medicine   Stephanie Saul, "Record Sales of Sleeping Pills Are Causing Worries," *New York Times*, February 7, 2006.

16. THE LAST PLACE YOU LOOK
Thyroid Low? Blood Pressure High? A Host of Common Midlife Disorders Pack a Cognitive Wallop

189 Lyme disease   Michelle Tauber, "A New Ending," *People Magazine*, November 3, 2003.

190 chronic fatigue syndrome   Mary A. Fischer, "You Think You're Tired," *O Magazine*, September 2006, 231–236.

191 complication of cardiopulmonary bypass surgery   Diederik van Dijk et al., "Cognitive Outcome After Off-Pump and On-Pump Coronary Artery Bypass Graft Surgery: A Randomized Trial," *Journal of the American Medical Association* 287 (2002): 1405–1412.

191 transient global amnesia   Carole Tanzer Miller, "Oh No! What Happened to the Afterglow? Some People Lapse into Amnesia After Sex," HealthScoutNews.com, June 24, 2003, http://www.geometry.net/detail/health_conditions/transient_global_amnesia_page_no_4.html.

191 the brain is the last in line   Antonio Convit, interview by the author, March 2, 2004.

192 "if someone is fat, it may affect [his] brain."   Cary Groner, "Researchers Gain Insight into Link Between Weight and Dementia," *Applied Neurology*, March 2006; viewed online at http://appneurology.com/showArticle.jhtml?articleId=184417526.

192 American men are overweight   Harvey B. Simon, "Longevity: The Ultimate Gender Gap," *Scientific American*, "The Science of Staying Young" special edition, June 2004.

192 "metabolic syndrome," "Link Between Cardiovascular Risk and Cognitive Decline," University of California, San Francisco press release, November 10, 2004.

192 body's ability to handle glucose, or blood sugar Convit interview.

192 blood glucose levels are too high "Heading Off the Diabetes Crisis," *Consumer Reports on Health*, August 2004.

193 There are no symptoms of impaired glucose tolerance Convit interview.

193 The glucose tolerance test requires an overnight fast Ibid.

193 People who have impaired glucose tolerance Ibid.

193 one in three American children Denise Grady, "Link Between Diabetes and Alzheimer's Disease Deepens," *New York Times*, July 17, 2006, F1.

194 American men (in addition to being overweight) are not regularly active Simon, "Longevity: The Ultimate Gender Gap."

194 In this chain reaction, insulin Groner, *Applied Neurology*.

195 Long-term insulin resistance Ibid.

195 Over 20 percent of adult Americans suffer "The Johns Hopkins White Paper Bulletins," *Memory*, 2005.

195 blood pressure dips "Higher Nighttime Blood Pressure Linked to Lower Cognitive Function," Newswise press release, November 6, 2005.

196 Risk factors for anemia Ben Harder, "Blood, Iron, and Gray Hair: Anemia in Old Age Is a Rising Concern," *Science News*, June 3, 2006, 346.

198 the thyroid is the gas pedal for every organ and cell "Memory Loss and Thyroid Function," Great Smokies Diagnostic Laboratory 2002, http://www.gdx.net/home/assessments/finddisease/memory/thyroid.html.

198 the brain uses thyroid-stimulating hormone Yodphat Krausz et al., "Regional Cerebral Blood Flow in Patients with Mild Hypothyroidism," *Journal of Nuclear Medicine* 45, no. 10 (2004): 1712–1715; "Cerebral Blood Flow and Glucose Metabolism in Hypothyroidism: A Positron Emission Tomography Study," *Journal of Clinical Endocrinology and Metabolism* 86, no. 8 (2001): 3864–3870.

198 Hypothyroidism results Kate Murphy, "For Thyroid Hormones, How Low Is Too Low?" *New York Times*, November 8, 2005.

199 mounting evidence that any TSH over 2.5 is abnormal Ibid.

199 Lowering the TSH range Ibid.

199 He'd written some books on thyroid and hormonal disorders Richard Shames, *Feeling Fat, Fuzzy or Frazzled? A 3-Step Program to Beat Hormone Havoc; Restore Thyroid, Adrenal, and Reproductive Balance; and Feel Better Fast* (New York: Hudson Street Press, 2005); *Thyroid Power: Ten Steps to Total Health* (New York: HarperCollins, 2002).

199 he looked and listened for over an hour Richard Shames, interview by the author, March 9, 2005.

201 synthetic T-4 (Synthroid) Joe and Terry Graedon, "Graedons' Guide to Thyroid Hormones," *The Peoples' Pharmacy*, www.peoplespharmacy.com.

201 I told him the news Richard Shames, interview by the author, April 6, 2005.

202 "But how's your memory?" Richard Shames, interview by the author, May 3, 2005.

17. STARING INTO THE EYE OF THE TIGER
Deep in the Grip of Alzheimer's Disease at the Age of Sixty, Joanna Graciously
Invites Us into Her World

204 we could meet each other in person   Dates of interviews with Joanna and Theo
May 4, 2005; April 2, 2006.

208 clinical trial of Neurochem's Alzhemed   "New Drug Alzhemed Shows Early
Promise Against Alzheimer's," Fisher Center for Alzheimer's Research Foun-
dation press release, November 4, 2003; "Neurochem Receives Third Positive
Recommendation from Independent Safety Review Board to Continue Phase
III Clinical Trial For Alzhemed," Neurochem press release, October 5, 2005.

208 Joanna would be entitled   Theo, e-mail to the author, August 3, 2006.

208 Forest Lab's Namenda   "The Johns Hopkins White Papers," *Memory*, 2005.

208 Namenda works by regulating levels of glutamate   Constantine Lyketsos, "The
11th Annual Update on the Treatment of Alzheimer's and Related Disorders:
Defining the Standard of Care," Hopkins White Paper Bulletins, Spring 2005
issue (April 22, 2005).

210 the COGNIshunt study   "Decreasing Toxins in Brain of Alzheimer's Patients
Keep Cognitive Deficits at Bay," University of Pennsylvania press release,
August 23, 2004.

210 Insulin and a related protein, IGF-1   Cary Groner, "Researchers Gain Insight into
Link Between Weight and Dementia," *Applied Neurology*, May 2006; Suzanne M.
de la Monte, "Insulin and Insulin-Like Growth Factor Expression and Function
Deteriorate with Progression of Alzheimer's Disease: Link to Brain Reductions in
Acetylcholine," *Journal of Alzheimer's Disease* 8, no. 3 (2005): 247–268.

210 insulin levels are nearly 80 percent lower   Ibid.

210 relationship between insulin, acetylcholine levels and Alzheimer's   Rebecca
Logsdon, "Spotlight on Research: Studies from the Memory Wellness Program
Lead to Greater Understanding of Insulin and Memory," *Dimensions*, Winter
2006; viewed at http://www.hopkinsmemory.com.

211 enlists the body's immune system to clean up the plaques and tangles   Scott
Hensley, "New Hope Seen for Vaccine for Alzheimer's," *Wall Street Journal*,
July 22, 2004.

211 AF267B, a disease-modifying compound   Kate Wong, "Drug Found to Reverse the Ravages of Alzheimer's in Mice," *Scientific American*, March 1, 2006.

211 intravenous immuglobulin therapy, called IVIg   "In Preliminary Study, New
York-Presbyterian/Weill Cornell Team Finds IVIg Therapy May Improve Cognitive Function in Alzheimer's Patients," Cornell press release, April 11, 2005.

211 IVIg has already passed the FDA's   Ibid.

212 neurons that produce acetylcholine   Mark Tuszynski, interview by the author,
October 6, 2006.

213 PTSD and depression increased the risk of developing Alzheimer's disease   Douglas Bremner, *Does Stress Damage the Brain? Understanding Trauma-
Related Disorders from a Mind Body Perspective* (New York: Norton, 2002).

214 Joanna's condition was declining visibly. Theo, e-mail to the author, October 16, 2005.

18. DO YOU REALLY WANT TO KNOW?
As Opportunities for Early Assessment and Intervention Become Available, Will You Embrace Them?

218 "'trouble with words'" Ronald Peterson, interview by the author, July 14, 2004.

218 "We need more diagnostic accuracy" John Trojanowski, interview by the author, October 10, 2005.

219 Alzheimer's Disease Neuroimaging Initiative Richard J. Hodes, "Public Funding for Alzheimer Disease."

219 foolproof method of diagnosing Alzheimer's John Trojanowski, interview by the author, April 27, 2004.

219 hunt for Alzheimer's biomarkers John Q. Trojanowski, "Searching for the Biomarkers of Alzheimer's," *Practical Neurology* 3 December 2004: 30–34.

219 "looking for diagnostic laboratory tests" Trojanowski interview.

219 "We need a test that is age-blind" Trojanowski interview.

219 A panel of markers Trojanowski interview.

219 already found a few promising biomarkers Trojanowski interview; "Taking Action to Prevent Mild Cognitive Deficit after 60 May Hinge on Knowing Levels of Factor in Blood," Boston University press release, September 27, 2005.

219 most promising markers exist in cerebrospinal fluid Kaj Blennow, "Use of CSF Biomarkers in Clinical Diagnosis and to Monitor Treatment Effects," paper presented at the 9th International Geneva/Springfield Symposium on Advances in Alzheimer Therapy, April 20, 2006.

219 "we'll find what we need" Trojanowski interview.

220 image-analysis technique Apoorva Mandavilli, "The Amyloid Code," *Nature Medicine*, 12, no. 7 (2006): 747–751.

220 "we can show with great accuracy who will develop Alzheimer's disease" Mony de Leon, interview by the author, March 2, 2004.

220 "We're clearly not there yet." Trojanowski interview.

221 "It's a great-looking hippocampus" Mony de Leon, interview by the author, May 25, 2005.

221 method of assessment that looks very promising Laurie Tarkan, "Predicting Alzheimer's Is More Wish Than Reality," *New York Times*, October 25, 2005; Marjorie Shaffer, "New Analysis of a Standard Brain Test May Help Predict Dementia," NYU Research: A Digest of Research News from New York University, Fall 2005.

222 The apolipoprotein gene "The Johns Hopkins White Paper Bulletins," *Memory*, 2005.

222 Everybody carries two copies of it, one from each parent Ibid.

222 In this particular gene, the alleles are called E2, E3 and E4 Ibid.

222 People who carry a single E4 variant   James Bakalar and Anthony L. Komaroff, "The Aging Brain: Old Genes, New Findings," *Newsweek*, January 17, 2005.

222 carry two copies of the E4 allele   "The Johns Hopkins White Paper Bulletins," *Memory*, 2005.

222 E4 carriers show symptoms of memory decline   Ibid.

222 ApoE is a susceptibility gene   Ibid.

222 Some people who carry double E4 alleles   www.alzheimers.org.

222 ApoE is a protein that helps shuttle cholesterol   G. William Rebeck et al., "Apolipoprotein E Receptor 2 Interactions with the N-Methyl-D-aspartate Receptor," *Journal of Biological Chemistry* 281, no. 6 (2006): 3425–3431.

222 It picks up lipids and other materials   Ibid.

222 E4 is a laggard   Ibid.

222 It increases the risk of diabetes   Bakalar and Komaroff, "The Aging Brain."

222 People who carry E4 and drink alcohol   Miia Kivipelto et al., "Alcohol Drinking in Middle Age and Subsequent Risk of Mild Cognitive Impairment and Dementia in Old Age: A Prospective Population-Based Study," *British Medical Journal*, September 4, 2004: 539–542.

223 supplementary estrogen notably improves learning   Roberta Diaz Brinton and Liqin Zhao, "Estrogen Receptor B as a Therapeutic Target for Promoting Neurogenesis and Preventing Neurodegeneration," *Drug Development Research* 66, no. 2 (2006): 103–107.

223 Individuals who carry the E4 variant   Daniel Michaelson et al., "Stimulation and Amyloid-B Mediated Activation of Apoptosis and Neurogenesis In-Vivo By Apolipoprotein E4," paper presented at the 9th Geneva/Springfield Symposium on Advances in Alzheimer Therapy, April 21, 2006.

223 Myelin, the fatty coating that protects axons   George Bartzokis, "Apolipoprotein E Genotype and Age-Related Myelin Breakdown in Healthy Individuals: Implications for Cognitive Decline and Dementia," *Archives of General Psychiatry* 63: January 2006, 57–62.

223 interfere with neurons' ability to make use of glucose   Yadong Huang et al., "Lipid- and Receptor-Binding Regions of Apolipoprotein E4 Fragments Act in Concert to Cause Mitochondrial Dysfunction and Neurotoxicity," *Proceedings of the National Academy of Science* 102, no. 51 (2005):18694–18699.

223 In PET imaging of cognitively normal subjects   "Changes Linked to Alzheimer's Examined," *The Associated Press*, December 16, 2003; Richard Caselli et al., "Preclinical Cognitive Decline in Late Middle-Aged Asymptomatic Apolipoprotein E-E4/4 Homozygotes: A Replication Study," *Journal of Neurological Sciences* 189 (2001): 93–98.

223 people who carried the E4 variant   Eric Reiman et al., "Preclinical Evidence of Alzheimer's Disease in Persons Homozygous for the E-4 Allele for Apolipoprotein E," *New England Journal of Medicine*, 334, no. 12 (1996): 752–758.

223 more frontal-lobe functional impairment   Richard Caselli et al., "A Distinctive Interraction Between Chronic Anxiety and Problem Solving in Asymptomatic

APOE e4 Homozygotes," *Journal of Neuropsychiatry and Clinical Neuroscience* 16 (August 2004): 320–329.

223 advised physicians against ordering the test   See http://www.nia.nih.gov/News AndEvents/PressReleases/PR19931107PossibleTargets.htm.

223 the risk of misunderstandings outweighs the potential benefits   Robert C. Green, "Risk Assessment for Alzheimer's Disease with Genetic Susceptibility Testing: Has the Moment Arrived?" *Alzheimer's Care Quarterly*, Summer 2002: 208–214.

224 Robert Green, a professor of neurology, genetics and epidemiology   Robert Green, interview by the author, March 9, 2004.

224 As the principal investigator and director of REVEAL   Ibid.

224 "We have all sorts of safety checks and balances in place"   Ibid.

224 "genotype does not determine"   Ibid.

224 powerful presymptomatic risk factor   Robert Green, e-mail to the author, September 8, 2006.

224 the protocol for REVEAL   Ibid.

225 "When a daughter comes in with the parent"   Ibid.

226 E4 carriers who'd experienced head trauma   J. A. R. Nicoll et al., "Association of APOE e4 and Cerebrovascular Pathology in Traumatic Brain Injury," *Journal of Neurology, Neurosurgery, and Psychiatry* 77 (2006): 363–366.

226 without a first-degree relative   Robert Green, e-mail to the author, August 8, 2004.

226 I'd need a diagnosis of unspecified dementia   Ibid.

226 Athena Diagnositics   See http://www.athenadiagnostics.com.

19. EMERGING TRIUMPHANT
How to Stockpile Neurons: The Habits of the Cognitively Well-Endowed

229 Five percent of people between the ages   Denise C. Park and Angela H. Gutchess, "Long-Term Memory and Aging: A Cognitive Neuroscience Perspective," in Roberto Cabeza, Lars Nyberg, and Denise C. Park, eds., *Cognitive Neuroscience of Aging: Linking Cognitive and Cerebral Aging* (New York: Oxford University Press, 2004), 218–245.

229 the father of learning and memory research   Eric Kandel, interview by the author, April 14, 2004.

230 studies how people develop "cognitive reserve"   Yaakov Stern, interview by the author, March 7, 2006.

230 "greater functional longevity"   Elkhonon Goldberg, *The Executive Brain: Frontal Lobes and the Civilized Mind* (New York: Oxford University Press, 2002).

231 involving concentration and multitasking   Park and Gutchess, "Long-Term Memory and Aging."

231 the case of Robert Wetherill   Lisa Melton, "How Brainpower Can Help You Cheat Old Age," *New Scientist*, December 17, 2005.

232 "high cognitive reserve might keep you"   Stern interview.

232 the greatest determinant of adult cognitive function   Marcus Richards et al., "Cognitive Ability in Childhood and Cognitive Decline in Midlife: Longitudinal Birth Cohort Study, *British Medical Journal* 328 (March 6, 2004): 552.

232 it would be interesting to track the cognitive health   Stern interview.

234 "a person's mind will grow crippled, hardened, sclerotic."   Simone de Beauvoir, *The Coming of Age* (New York: Putnam, 1972), 393.

234 those who pursue advanced degrees build additional resilience   Mellanie Springer, "The Relation Between Brain Activity During Memory Tasks and Years of Education in Young and Older Adults," *Neuropsychology* 19 (March 2005): 181–192.

235 the mind-enhancing benefits of motherhood. Katherine Ellison, *The Mommy Brain: How Motherhood Makes Us Smarter* (New York: Basic Books, 2005).

235 the greatest cognitive benefits derived   Podewils et al., "Physical Activity, APOE Genotype, and Dementia Risk. Findings from the Cardiovascular Health Cognition Study," *American Journal of Epidemiology* 161, no. 7 (2005): 639–651.

237 moved to Minneapolis   Charles Baxter, e-mail to the author, January 27, 2004.

237 I met the structure that temporarily contained him   Richard Lang, interview by the author, November 10, 2004.

239 elderly people who participated in aerobic fitness   A. F. Kramer et al., "Cardiovascular Fitness, Cortical Plasticity, and Aging," *Proceedings of the National Academy of Science* 101, no. 9 (2004): 3316–3321.

239 physical activity just twice a week   Miia Kivipelto, "Does Healthy Lifestyle Protect Against Dementia?" Paper presented at the 9th International Geneva/Springfield Symposium on Advances in Alzheimer Therapy, April 20, 2006.

239 mice that started exercising in old age   Henriette van Praag et al., "Exercise Enhances Learning and Hippocampal Neurogenesis in Aged Mice," *Journal of Neuroscience* 25, no. 38 (September 2005): 8680–8685.

239 I saw a picture in *Health* magazine of Nan Wiener   "Nan Wiener, Salsa Dancing," *Health*, June 2003, 119.

239 ballroom dancing reduced the risk   Joe Verghese et al., "Leisure Activities and the Risk of Dementia in the Elderly," *New England Journal of Medicine* 348 (June 19, 2003): 2508–2516.

240 she'd been dancing   Nan Wiener, interview by the author, March 11, 2005.

240 We agreed to meet in Sausalito, at Horizons   Ibid.

241 tango dancing   "Studies with Dancing, Computer Training, Show Ways to Maintain a Healthy Brain in Old Age," Posit Science press release, November 15, 2005.

242 the effect of individualized piano instruction   Jennifer Bugos et al., "The Effects of Individualized Piano Instruction on Executive Memory Functions in Older Adults (Ages 60–85)," paper presented at the 8th International Conference on Music Perception and Cognition, 2004.

243 She'd always wanted to be a doctor   Dawn Swanson, interview by the author, May 25, 2004.

246 people who solved crossword puzzles   Verghese et al., "Leisure Activities and the Risk of Dementia in the Elderly."

247 editor of the *New York Times* crossword puzzle   Will Shortz, interview by the author, January 25, 2006.

248 the *New York Times* Puzzle Forum message board   Follow link to Forum from http://www.nytimes.com/pages/crosswords/.

248 "I was forgetting birthdays"   Courtenay "Co" Crocker, e-mail to the author, January 25, 2006.

249 All the senses are tapped   Eric Nagourney, "Social Whirl May Help Keep the Mind Dancing," *New York Times*, October 29, 2002.

249 the importance of social involvement   Laura Fratiglioni et al., "Mental, Physical and Social Components in Common Leisure Activities in Old Age in Relation to Dementia: Findings from the Kungsholmen Project," paper presented at the Alzheimer's Association 9th International Conference on Alzheimer's Disease and Related Disorders, Philadelphia, July 17–22, 2004. Abstract published in *Neurobiology of Aging* 25, S2: S313, July 2004.

249 "social interaction is way down"   Lawrence Katz, interview by the author, April 22, 2004.

250 "You need a plan"   Edward Hallowell, *CrazyBusy: Overstretched, Overbooked, and About to Snap!* (New York: Ballantine, 2006), 39.

250 "live meetings have been replaced"   Ibid., 82.

250 71 percent of seniors   "Studies with Dancing, Computer Training."

250 to the house in Larkspur   Zvi and Marjorie Danenberg, interview by the author, October 6, 2005.

CONCLUSION

256 "Asked how they would describe their memories"   Thomas Crook, interview by the author, October 14, 2004.

SELECTED BIBLIOGRAPHY

. . .

I read a great many books that did not necessarily make it into the direct references, but they informed my thinking nonetheless.

Ackerman, Diane. *An Alchemy of the Mind: The Marvel and Mystery of the Brain.* New York: Scribner, 2004.

Aldridge, Susan. *Magic Molecules: How Drugs Work.* London: Cambridge University Press, 1998.

Angier, Natalie. *Woman: An Intimate Geography.* Boston: Houghton Mifflin, 1999.

Archibald, Robert. *A Place to Remember: Using History to Build Community.* Walnut Creek, CA: Altamira Press, 1999.

Barondes, Samuel H. *Better than Prozac: Creating the Next Generation of Psychiatric Drugs.* New York: Oxford University Press, 2003.

Baxter, Charles, ed. *The Business of Memory: The Art of Remembering in an Age of Forgetting.* Saint Paul, MN: Graywolf Press, 1999.

Borges, Jorge Luis. "Funes, the Memorious," in *Ficciones.* New York: Knopf, 1993.

Bourtchouladze, Rusiko. *Memories Are Made of This: How Memory Works in Humans and Animals.* New York: Columbia University Press, 2002.

Breggin, Peter, and David Cohen. *Your Drug May Be Your Problem: How and Why to Stop Taking Psychiatric Medications.* Cambridge, MA: Perseus, 1999.

Bremner, Douglas J. *Does Stress Damage the Brain? Understanding Trauma-Related Disorders from a Mind-Body Perspective.* New York: Norton, 2002.

Calvin, William H. *A Brain for All Seasons: Human Evolution and Abrupt Climate Change.* Chicago: University of Chicago Press, 2002.

Clark, Andy. *Natural-Born Cyborgs: Minds, Technologies, and the Future of Human Intelligence.* New York: Oxford University Press, 2003.

Collins, Billy. *Questions About Angels*. Pittsburgh: University of Pittsburgh Press, 1991.

d'Assigny, Marius. *The Art of Memory*. New York: AMS Press, 1985.

de Beauvoir, Simone. *The Coming of Age*, New York: Putnam, 1972.

de Graaf, John. *Affluenza: The All-Consuming Epidemic*. San Francisco: Berrett-Koehler Publishers, 2001.

Diamond, Jared M. *The Third Chimpanzee: The Evolution and Future of the Human Animal*. New York: HarperCollins, 1992.

Draaisma, Douwe. *Metaphors of Memory: A History of Ideas About the Mind*. Cambridge, UK: Cambridge University Press, 2000.

Ellison, Katherine. *The Mommy Brain: How Motherhood Makes Us Smarter*. New York: Basic Books, 2005.

Engel, Susan. *Context Is Everything: The Nature of Memory*. New York: Henry Holt, 2000.

Forty, Adrian, and Susanne Kuchler, eds. *The Art of Forgetting*. Oxford: Berg, 1999.

Fukuyama, Francis. *Our Posthuman Future: Consequences of the Biotechnology Revolution*. New York: Farrar Straus & Giroux, 2002.

Gleick, James. *What Just Happened: A Chronicle from the Information Frontier*. New York: Pantheon, 2002.

Glenmullen, Joseph. *The Antidepressant Solution: A Step-by-Step Guide to Safely Overcoming Antidepressant Withdrawal, Dependence, and "Addiction."* New York: Free Press, 2004.

Goldberg, Elkhonon. *The Executive Brain: The Frontal Lobes and the Civilized Mind*. New York: Oxford University Press, 2001.

——. *The Wisdom Paradox: How Your Mind Can Grow Stronger as Your Brain Grows Older*. New York: Gotham, 2005.

Gordon, Barry. *Intelligent Memory: Improve Your Memory No Matter What Your Age*. New York: Viking Adult, 2003.

Gruneberg, Michael, and Peter Morris, eds. *Aspects of Memory*, 2d ed. Vol. 1: *The Practical Aspects*. London: Routledge, 1992.

Gullette, Margaret Morganroth. *Aged by Culture*. Chicago: University of Chicago Press, 2004.

——. *Declining to Decline: Cultural Combat and the Politics of the Midlife*. Charlottesville, VA: University Press of Virginia, 1997.

Hallowell, Edward M. *CrazyBusy: Overstretched, Overbooked, and About to Snap! Strategies for Coping in a World Gone ADD*. New York: Ballantine, 2006.

——. *Delivered from Distraction: Getting the Most out of Life with Attention Deficit Disorder*. New York: Ballantine, 2005.

—— and John J. Ratey. *Driven to Distraction: Recognizing and Coping with Attention Deficit Disorder from Childhood Through Adulthood*. New York: Pantheon, 1994.

Hawkins, Jeff, and Sandra Blakeslee. *On Intelligence*. New York: Times Books, 2004.

Honore, Carl. *In Praise of Slowness: How a Worldwide Movement Is Challenging the Cult of Speed.* San Francisco: HarperSanFrancisco, 2004.

Johnson, Steven. *Mind Wide Open: Your Brain and the Neuroscience of Everyday Life*. New York: Scribner, 2004.

Kabat-Zinn, Jon. *Full Catastrophe Living: Using the Wisdom of Your Body and Mind to Face Stress, Pain, and Illness*. New York: Delacorte Press, 1990.

Kammen, Michael. *Mystic Chords of Memory: The Transformation of Tradition in American Culture*. New York: Knopf, 1991.

Katz, Lawrence C., and Manning Rubin. *Keep Your Brain Alive—83 Neurobic Exercises*. New York: Workman, 1998.

Kemper, Susan, and Reinhold Kliegl, eds. *Constraints on Language: Aging, Grammar, and Memory*. Boston: Kluwer Academic Publishers, 1999.

Khalsa, Dharma Singh, with Cameron Stauth. *Brain Longevity: The Breakthrough Medical Program That Improves Your Mind and Your Memory*. New York: Warner Books, 1997.

Kimura, Deborah. *Sex and Cognition*. Cambridge, MA: MIT Press, 2000.

Lerner, Harriet. *The Dance of Anger*. New York: HarperCollins, 1985.

McEwen, Bruce, with Elizabeth Norton Lasley. *The End of Stress as We Know It*. Washington, DC: National Academies Press, 2002.

McGaugh, James. *Memory and Emotion: The Making of Lasting Memories*. New York: Columbia University Press, 2003.

McKhann, Guy, and Marilyn Albert. *Keep Your Brain Young: The Complete Guide to Physical and Emotional Health and Longevity*. New York: Wiley, 2002.

Perlmutter, David. *The Better Brain Book*. New York: Riverhead, 2004.

Plant, Sadie. *Writing on Drugs*. New York: Farrar, Straus & Giroux, 1999.

Postman, Neil. *Technopoly*. New York: Knopf, 1992.

Roach, Mary. *The Curious Lives of Human Cadavers*. New York: Norton, 2003.

Rupp, Rebecca. *Committed to Memory: How We Remember and Why We Forget*. New York: Crown, 1997.

Sapolsky, Robert M. *Monkeyluv and Other Essays on Our Lives as Animals*. New York: Scribner, 2005.

———. *A Primate's Memoir*. New York: Scribner, 2001.

———. *Why Zebras Don't Get Ulcers: A Guide to Stress, Stress-Related Diseases, and Coping*. New York: Freeman, 1994.

Schacter, Daniel L. *Searching for Memory: The Brain, the Mind, and the Past*. New York: Basic Books, 1996.

———. *The Seven Sins of Memory: How the Mind Forgets and Remembers*. Boston: Houghton Mifflin, 2001.

Schwartz, Jeffrey, and Sharon Begley. *The Mind and the Brain: Neuroplasticity and the Power of Mental Force*. New York: Regan Books, 2002.

Shames, Richard. *Feeling Fat, Fuzzy or Frazzled? A 3-Step Program to Beat Hormone Havoc; Restore Thyroid, Adrenal, and Reproductive Balance; and Feel Better Fast*. New York: Hudson Street Press, 2005.

———. *Thyroid Power: Ten Steps to Total Health*. New York: HarperCollins, 2002.

Shenk, David. *Data Smog: Surviving the Information Glut*. New York: HarperEdge, 1997.

———. *The Forgetting: Alzheimer's: Portrait of an Epidemic*. New York: Anchor Books, 2003.

Shweder, Richard A., ed. *Welcome to Middle Age! (And Other Cultural Fictions)*. Chicago: University of Chicago Press, 1998.

Siegel, Daniel. *The Developing Mind: Toward a Neurobiology of Interpersonal Experience.* New York: Guilford Press, 1999.

—— and Mary Hartzell. *Parenting from the Inside Out.* New York: Tarcher, 2003.

Skloot, Floyd. *In the Shadow of Memory.* Lincoln, NE: Bison Books, 2004.

Small, Gary, and Gigi Vorgan. *The Longevity Bible: 8 Essential Strategies for Keeping Your Mind Sharp and Your Body Young.* New York: Hyperion, 2006.

——. *The Memory Bible: An Innovative Strategy for Keeping Your Brain Young.* New York: Hyperion, 2002.

—— and Gigi Vorgan. *The Memory Prescription: Dr. Gary Small's 14-Day Plan to Keep Your Brain and Body Young.* New York: Hyperion, 2004.

Solomon, Andrew. *The Noonday Demon: An Atlas of Depression.* New York: Scribner, 2001.

Squire, Larry R., and Eric R. Kandel. *Memory: From Mind to Molecules.* New York: Scientific American Library, 1999.

Stacey, Michelle. *The Fasting Girl: A True Victorian Medical Mystery.* New York: Tarcher/Penguin, 2002.

Sternberg, Robert J., ed. *Wisdom: Its Nature, Origins and Development.* Cambridge, UK: Cambridge University Press, 1990.

Stoler, Diane Roberts, and Barbara Albers Hill. *Coping with Mild Traumatic Brain Injury.* New York: Avery, 1998.

Vaillant, George E. *Aging Well: Surprising Guideposts to a Happier Life from the Landmark Harvard Study of Adult Development.* New York: Time Warner, 2002.

Warga, Claire. *Menopause and the Mind: The Complete Guide to Coping with the Cognitive Effects of Perimenopause and Menopause Including: Memory Loss, Foggy Thinking, and Verbal Slips.* New York: Touchstone, 2000.

Warnock, Mary. *Memory.* London: Faber and Faber, 1987.

Wise, Anna. *The High-Performance Mind: Mastering Brainwaves for Insight, Healing, and Creativity.* New York: Tarcher, 1997.

INDEX

. . .

301